Contents

A Word from the Author

O ne of the more rewarding aspects of writing a book of games and puzzles is hearing from so many of you— the readers. Your emails and letters remind me that for many people, games can be much more than just an amusing diversion.

Games often bring people together. One family in the Midwest wrote that they had "the best Thanksgiving ever" when four generations of women (mother, daughter, granddaughter, and great-granddaughter) spent hours after dinner "playing the games and laughing up a storm."

Games can also offer a welcome distraction during difficult times. A man in upstate New York was going through weeks of surgery, chemotherapy, and radiation. His wife wrote to thank me. "Your books got us through," she said, "I don't know what we would have done without them."

I've heard from teachers who use my games to start each day with a little fun; from speech therapists who use them to help victims of stroke or head injuries regain their voices. And I hear from so many adult children of parents who are in the early- to mid-stages of dementia. They struggle, not always successfully, to find ways to communicate with Mom or Dad. Playing carefully

299 *on-the-go* games & puzzles to keep your brain young.

NANCY LINDE

WORKMAN PUBLISHING • NEW YORK

Library of Congress Cataloging-in-Publication Data is available.

ISBN 978-1-5235-0647-7

Design by Galen Smith
Cover: Copyright © Carlos Gardel/Adobe Stock (head silhouette), Gst/Shutterstock.com (brain).

Workman books are available at special discounts when purchased in bulk for premiums and sales promotions as well as for fund-raising or educational use. Special editions or book excerpts can also be created to specification. For details, contact the Special Sales Director at the address below, or send an email to specialmarkets@workman.com.

Workman Publishing Co., Inc.
225 Varick Street
New York, NY 10014-4381
workman.com

WORKMAN is a registered trademark of Workman Publishing Co., Inc.

Printed in the United States of America

First printing November 2019

10 9 8 7 6 5 4 3 2 1

chosen games can briefly recapture an easier time and provide some moments of shared joy.

Games Are More Than Just an Amusing Diversion

The benefits of games go even further. Recent research shows that people who are mentally active in their later years (solving brain games, learning to play a musical instrument, taking up chess, or even learning a foreign language) are more mentally sharp, cognitively agile, and have better memory functions. In the same way that physical exercise postpones and reduces loss of muscle mass and increases physical flexibility, mental exercise sharpens memory, concentration, and *mental* flexibility.

How can you use this book to help your brain? I'll get to that in a minute, but first a word of caution. Games are just one part of a healthy lifestyle for a healthy brain. Nothing beats the basics, which include eating properly, getting enough sleep, and getting some physical exercise every day . . . you know the drill. But one thing is certain—of all the things you do to stay healthy, games are likely to be the most fun!

How to Use This Book

If you simply like word games and brain puzzles, then dig right in and start playing. But if you are also a person who wants to improve your memory and sharpen your mind, read on. Because this is not just a book of games, it is also a rigorous exercise workout to keep your brain in tip-top shape.

What follows is a summary of the same good advice that Philip D. Harvey, PhD, provided in my previous books (*399 Games, Puzzles, and Trivia Challenges Specially Designed to Keep Your Brain Young* and its follow-up volume *417 More Games, Puzzles, and Trivia Challenges Specially Designed to Keep Your Brain Young*). It will help you identify which of your own cognitive functions need a good workout and suggests some of the games that will help.

Just keep in mind that a fitness routine for the brain works just like an exercise program for the body. If you want to build up your biceps, you might start lifting weights; if you want to tighten your abs, you would probably do abdominal crunches. Applying that same logic to the brain, if you want to improve your *long-term memory*, you should choose games that are challenging for you and that stretch those cognitive "muscles." Or, if you'd like to process your thoughts faster and with more clarity, then you should look for games that address *processing speed*.

Six Key Cognitive Skills That Are Vulnerable in Normal Aging

Living normally and independently in the world requires many different cognitive abilities. Some, such as basic perception (sight, hearing, etc.) and sensory processes (touch, taste, etc.), usually don't change much in normal aging. Other cognitive functions are more vulnerable. A few years ago, we worked closely with Dr. Harvey to identify the key mental functions that are more likely than others to change with age. They are:

- Long-term memory
- Working memory
- Executive functioning
- Attention to detail
- Multitasking
- Processing speed

Let's take a closer look at each of those cognitive functions—the symptoms that frequently occur when age-related deterioration has taken place, and some of the games to look for that work specifically on that mental skill. You'll note that throughout the book we have labeled each game with the cognitive skill (or skills) that it primarily exercises.

1. LONG-TERM MEMORY. Long-term memory is exactly what the label implies—the ability to remember people, objects, or events that occurred in the distant past. If you have noticed occasional memory lapses, such as details from a long-ago vacation or the name of your favorite high school teacher, you should play games that exercise your long-term memory skills. Three good examples include: **Counting Syllables**, **Run the Alphabet**, and **Two By Three**.

2. WORKING MEMORY. Also called functional short-term memory, working memory is a basic mental skill. It's important for both learning and carrying out many everyday tasks. It enables the brain to briefly hold new information while it's needed in the short term. Working memory is in operation when you keep in mind the steps of a recipe while cooking a favorite family meal or going to the grocery store for four or five items without having to make a list. Games that boost your working memory skills include: **Double Trouble**, **Give Me a Word That . . .**, and **What's the Word?**.

3. EXECUTIVE FUNCTIONING. Executive functioning is a critical cognitive skill for everyday life. Without it, your life would be an unorganized mess. It involves solving problems by using information you already possess to work out novel solutions to a task or problem. If, for example, you are finding it more challenging to get organized and to accomplish routine tasks (such as running your weekend errands) efficiently or, if you find it hard to get out the door with everything you need (keys, phone, glasses), you should shape up your executive functioning skills. Three examples of fun ways to do that include **Fill In the Letters**, **Is or Isn't?**, and **Odd Man Out**.

4. ATTENTION TO DETAIL. The process of absorbing small details when learning new information requires the ability to concentrate and stay focused. If you're finding it hard to follow instructions when setting up or using new technology (such as a microwave oven or a DVD player), or if you have to study a subway map again and again to figure out how to get from point A to point B, or if you are having problems navigating a website to purchase an item or fill a prescription, you may need to play games that exercise your focus and concentration skills. Three examples of games that improve your attention to detail are **Change a Letter**, **Sentence Sleuth**, and **Wacky Wordy**.

5. MULTITASKING. Multitasking is a modern word that basically means doing more than one task at a time. Do you find yourself avoiding telephone "meetings" because you can't talk, listen, and take notes at the same time? Do you have trouble operating multiple controls in the car (radio, wipers, lights) while you are driving? Or do you need complete silence around you in order to read a book or work on your computer? If any of those symptoms apply to you, try games such as **Hidden Quotation**, **Making Connections**, and **Word Rebus** that focus on multitasking skills.

6. PROCESSING SPEED. This refers to the speed at which your brain processes information, which includes being mentally fast enough to keep up with conversations, follow the plot of television programs or movies, and complete tasks efficiently. If you have noticed that it takes longer for you to get simple tasks done, or if you need people to repeat things because you could not keep up, you may need to upgrade your processing speed skills. Any game that imposes a time limit, such as **Griddle**, **Run the Alphabet**, and **Tongue Twisters** is a good way to improve processing speed.

It's time for those on the go to get going . . .

What's particularly helpful about this book is that it was designed for people on the go. You don't have to carve out time to get your cognitive exercise in. This book is easy to carry (it fits into most purses or briefcases) and the games are short. Just take it with you wherever you go, and you can exercise your brain while you're waiting at the dentist's office, riding on the subway, watching your grandchildren at the playground, in line to get your driver's license renewed . . . the list is endless. And make sure you have fun while you keep your brain fit and fabulous.

CHAPTER ONE

Easy Does It

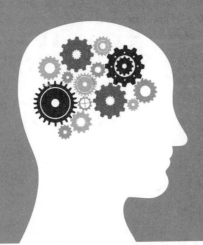

Is or Isn't?

In this game, you have to find the one item in each list that is—or isn't—what we say it is . . . or isn't.

1. Which actor is . . . in the 1997 movie *Titanic*?
   a. Tom Cruise   **b.** Leonardo DiCaprio
   c. Brad Pitt   **d.** Emma Thompson

2. Which dish isn't . . . Indian food?
   a. Samosa   **b.** Rogan josh
   c. Moolash   **d.** Biryani

3. Which name isn't . . . the name of a real baseball player?
   a. Vida Blue   **b.** Oil Can Boyd
   c. Coco Crisp   **d.** Maple Tree Wilson

4. Which city isn't . . . in Europe?
   a. Budapest   **b.** Baghdad
   c. Helsinki   **d.** Prague

Answers on page 314

What a Pair!

We provide half of a familiar word pairing. Can you come up with the other half?

1. Wit and _____

2. Bits and _____

3. _____ and cry

4. _____ and key

5. Part and _____

6. Rules and _____

Answers on page 314

Stinky Pinky

Each Stinky Pinky answer contains two words that rhyme. Can you figure out what the answer is from an offbeat definition? For example, the answer to the clue *Mrs. Onassis's tan pants* is *Jackie's khakis.*

1. A science research room for a leggy crustacean

2. A very bad smell in Paris

3. A small fake horse

4. A gloomy father

5. Hilarious currency

Answers on page 314

Word Rebus

multitasking,
attention to detail,
executive functioning

Each picture rebus represents a word. Pay close attention to the plus and minus signs to know which sound to add or remove.

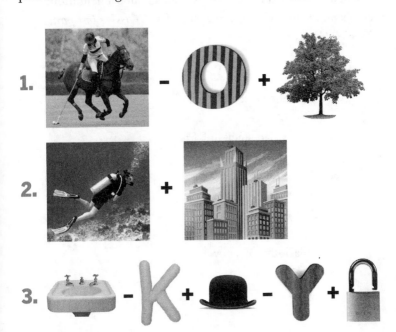

Answers on page 314

What's the Word?

working memory, attention to detail, executive functioning

Identify the missing letters that complete each row of words. For example, given the clues: _ _ _ **NERS**, **AL**_ _ _ **AC**, **HU**_ _ _, _ _ _ **SION**, the correct answer is *MAN (Manners, Almanac, Human, Mansion)*. *Note: All missing letters will form a three-letter word.*

VA _ _ _	COL _ _ _ E	SO _ _ _	HO _ _ _ AY
TH _ _ _	P _ _ _ ATE	_ _ _ OT	AC _ _ _ AT
_ _ _ ROOM	BOM _ _ _	CLIM _ _ _	STAB _ _ _
_ _ _ THER	_ _ _ TRY	_ _ _ CREAS	OCCU _ _ _ T

Answers on page 314

Run the Alphabet

From *Annex* to *Zax*, we're looking for a WORD THAT CONTAINS THE LETTER X for each letter of the alphabet. This game is a better brain booster if you put a two- or three-minute timer on it.

A_____   H_____   O_____   V_____

B_____   I_____   P_____   W_____

C_____   J_____   Q_____   X_____

D_____   K_____   R_____   Y *(none)*

E_____   L_____   S_____   Z *(obscure)*

F_____   M_____   T_____

G_____   N_____   U_____

Answers on page 314

ACRONYM ALPHABET

long-term memory, working memory

What do these common acronyms stand for?

1. DVM _____

2. ERA _____

3. FLOTUS _____

4. POV _____

5. VIN _____

6. OED _____

Answers on page 315

HIDDEN
QUOTATION

Cross out all words on the next page as instructed below. Then rearrange the remaining words (those that were not crossed out) to reveal a clever quotation.

1. Cross out all three-syllable words.

2. Cross out all musical instruments.

3. Cross out all animals.

4. Cross out all colors.

5. Cross out all cities.

long-term memory,
working memory,
attention to detail,
executive functioning

REGRET	CRIMSON	FROM	JUST
AREA	LONDON	LION	DRUM
GUITAR	LEARN	DON'T	GRAY
THE	IRONING	SEOUL	FLUTE
YAK	BOSTON	FROG	PAST
ECRU	IT	CELLO	AROMA

Quotation:

_____

_____

_____

Answers on page 315

Homonyms

long-term memory, attention to detail, executive functioning

Homonyms are two or more words that are pronounced the same but have different meanings and/or spellings (*to, two, too*). Given two definitions, you need to provide the homonyms, and spell them correctly.

1. A long cry of pain, grief, or anger; and a marine mammal

   _____   _____

2. An animal hunted for food; and to appeal to God

   _____   _____

3. To cause liquid to flow from a container; and a tiny opening in the skin

   _____   _____

4. A proboscis; and has information

   _____   _____

5. A person who claims to be able to predict the future; and a financial gain

   _____   _____

Answers on page 315

Riddle Me This

Classic riddles like this one are easier to solve if you think outside the box.

· · · · · · · · · · · · · · · · · · ·

Where does Christmas come before Thanksgiving?

· · · · · · · · · · · · · · · · · · ·

Answer on page 315

What's the Animal?

All the answers in this game are two-word idioms or phrases that contain the name of an animal. We provide the first word. Can you come up with the animal?

1. Cash _____

2. Eager _____

3. Grease _____

4. Silly _____

5. Spring _____

6. Dirty _____

Answers on page 315

Counting Syllables

long-term memory,
multitasking,
processing speed,
executive functioning

Come up with the answers to these questions, syllable by syllable. Put a one-minute timer on each question and you'll get a better brain workout.

1. Name the only US president with a four-syllable last name.

2. Name four fruits with one-syllable names.

3. Name three types of wood/trees with two-syllable names.

4. Name six world countries that have two-syllable names.

Answers on page 315

DOUBLE TROUBLE

Given a list of words such as *knuckle*, *moth*, and *basket*, can you find the one word that follows each of them to make a compound word or two-word phrase? For the example words above, the correct answer is *ball* (*knuckleball, mothball,* and *basketball*). *Note: The first letter of each answer is provided in a hint below . . . but try not to use it unless you're really stuck!*

1. Holy, Mineral, Spring

_____

3. Cow, Golden, Cover

_____

2. Odd, Wrong, Rational

_____

4. Egg, Figure, Letter

_____

(Hints: 1-W, 2-N, 3-G, 4-H)

Answers on page 315

Making Connections

multitasking, attention to detail, executive functioning

Given six words in the grid, can you find the three pairs that belong together and explain why each is a pair?

ZIP	DASH
ESCORT	NADA
PINTO	COLON

In the sample above, one pair is *Escort* and *Pinto*, which are both Ford car models. Another pair is *Zip* and *Nada*, which both mean *nothing*. And *Dash* and *Colon* are both punctuation marks.

GINGRICH	JUNK
BOBBY	BLITZER
KNEE	FAST

Pair_____   Theme _____

Pair_____   Theme _____

Pair_____   Theme _____

Answers on page 315

One-Minute Madness

How many DANCES (of any type) can you name in one minute?

_____

_____

_____

_____

_____

_____

_____

_____

_____

_____

_____

Answers on page 316

Change a Letter

Change the three given words into new words by replacing one letter—without rearranging any of the existing letters. For example: PLAY, SNAIL, WAIST can be changed to P<u>R</u>AY, SNA<u>R</u>L, W<u>R</u>IST. You can change any one of the existing letters, but you must use the same replacement letter for all three words.

1. Flask, Way, Pour _____ _____ _____

2. Umpire, Omit, Diving _____ _____ _____

3. Gym, Fly, Onion _____ _____ _____

4. Bring, Thin, Mango _____ _____ _____

Answers on page 316

Wacky Wordy

The arrangement of the letters in the frame is a clue to the answer. For example, if the word *school* were placed high up in the frame, the answer would be *high school*. Or if the phrase *easy pieces* occurred five times in the frame, the answer would be *five easy pieces*.

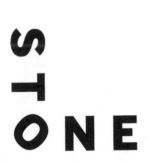

Answer on page 316

WORD TOWER

Build a tower of words that begins with the letters NO by increasing the number of letters in each consecutive word by one (example for the letters NO: NOT, NOON, NORTH, and so on). You cannot just add an S to a word already used, and no proper nouns are allowed. If you come up with words longer than eight letters, you're a Word Tower pro! *This game is a better brain booster if you put a one- or two-minute time limit on it.*

1. NO

2. NO __

3. NO __ __

4. NO __ __ __

5. NO __ __ __ __

6. NO __ __ __ __ __

7. NO __ __ __ __ __ __

8. NO __ __ __ __ __ __ __

Answers on page 316

JINGLES & SLOGANS

Finish the jingle or advertising slogan, and then name the product or company.

1. "Melts in your _____."

_____

2. "We'll leave the _____."

_____

3. "All the news that's _____."

_____

4. "When it absolutely, _____."

_____

5. "The happiest place _____."

_____

Answers on page 316

Fill In the Letters

long-term memory, attention to detail, processing speed, executive functioning

Fill in the blank spaces with letters to make common English words. (No proper nouns are allowed.) For example, the clue __ **a t** yields twelve answers: *Bat, Cat, Eat, Fat, Hat, Mat, Oat, Pat, Rat, Sat, Tat, Vat. Note: The number in parentheses indicates how many common English words we found.* For a better cognitive workout, put a one-minute timer on each puzzle below.

1. _ R _ T   (8)

2. D _ I _ Y   (6)

Answers on page 316

Common Bonds

long-term memory,
multitasking,
attention to detail

Find the common bond (or theme) among three very different pictures.

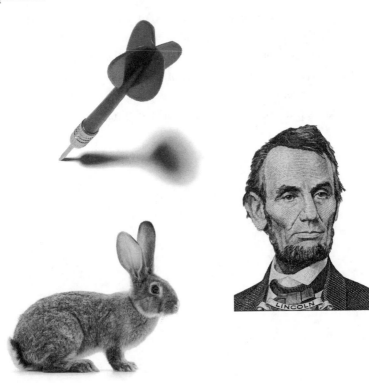

Answer on page 316

Four Tricky Tongue Twisters!

Repeat each tongue twister three times quickly and out loud, without making a mistake.

Greek grapes

Irish wristwatch

Willy's real rear wheel

Crisp crusts crunch and crackle

FINE
Words

Every word in this list is missing the letters **F-I-N-E**. Can you put those letters back (in any order) in the spaces below to reveal a common English word?

1. K __ __ __ __

2. BE __ __ __ __ T

3. CO __ __ __ D __

4. __ __ FTE __ __

5. ID __ __ T __ __ Y

6. O __ F __ __ S __ VE

Answers on page 316

Order, Please!

Given a list of three or four items, your job is to rearrange them in the order called for in the question.

1. Put these structures in order by height, starting with the tallest:

    _____ Statue of Liberty

    _____ Golden Gate Bridge

    _____ Eiffel Tower

2. Put these inventions in order of the year they were invented, starting with the earliest:

    _____ Elevator

    _____ Telephone

    _____ Telescope

Answers on page 317

SAY WHAT?

Saul loves sayings and proverbs … but he can never remember them correctly. Can you fix his mistakes to reveal the correct saying? For example, Saul might say: "Humans who reside in clear, vitreous residences ought not to hurl small rocks." But the correct saying is: "People who live in glass houses should not throw stones."

1. "Devotion compels the earth to spin on its axis."

   _____

   _____

2. "Mendicants are not able to be selectors."

   _____

   _____

3. "If you are unable to behave properly, use caution."

   _____

   _____

4. "Giggling and guffawing is the finest pharmaceutical product."

   _____

   _____

5. "There is no function in whipping an expired Appaloosa."

   _____

   _____

Answers on page 317

Animal Watching

These are not animals we see every day. Can you identify them?

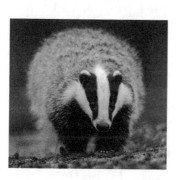

A.

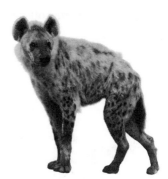

B.

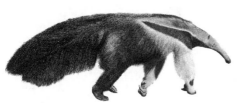

C.

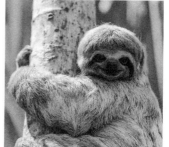

D.

Answers on page 317

Riddle
Me This

Classic riddles like this one are easier to solve if you think outside the box.

. . . .

What is more useful when it is broken?

. . . .

Answer on page 317

DOWN TO THE WIRE

long-term memory, working memory, processing speed

Put back the word or words that complete each expression. This is a better brain booster if you complete all the questions in one minute.

1. _____ to the music

2. _____ to the ground

3. _____ to the moon

4. _____ to the top

5. _____ to the wheel

Answers on page 317

EIGHTS & Fours

Can you make one eight-letter word and two four-letter words from the scrambled letters below?

1.

C D D R V E I O

_ _ _ _ _ _ _ _

_ _ _ _

_ _ _ _

2.

F G L N T A I O

_ _ _ _ _ _ _ _

_ _ _ _

_ _ _ _

Answers on page 317

Pictures & People

By combining one picture and one first name, can you come up with the full names of six famous people? *Note: The spelling may not always be exact, but the pronunciation will always be correct.*

PETER	EMILY	JOEY
AL	LARRY	JOAN

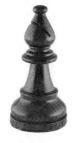 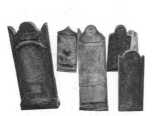 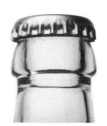

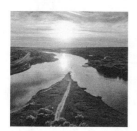 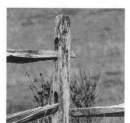 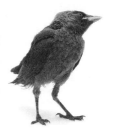

Answers on page 317

Griddle

Find as many words with four or more connected letters as you can in two minutes. The letters must touch either vertically, horizontally, or diagonally. You cannot skip or jump across letters, and you cannot use the same letter twice in one word. For example, to make the word *loyal*, you must have two Ls in the grid. Proper nouns are not allowed.

U	T	D	N
D	E	E	N
E	T	O	M
U	A	N	I

_____   _____   _____

_____   _____   _____

_____   _____   _____

_____   _____   _____

_____   _____   _____

_____   _____   _____

_____   _____   _____

_____   _____   _____

_____   _____   _____

_____   _____   _____

_____   _____   _____

_____   _____   _____

_____   _____   _____

_____   _____   _____

_____   _____   _____

Answers on page 317

Endings & Beginnings

In this game, we provide the first half of one compound word or two-word phrase and the second half of another. Can you come up with the one word that completes both? *Note: The first letter of each answer is provided in a hint below . . . but try not to use it unless you're really stuck!*

1. April _____ Proof

2. Touch _____ Town

3. Cottage _____ Cloth

4. Double _____ Word

5. Slap _____ Shift

OPPOSITES
ATTRACT

Rearrange the letters of each word provided to reveal a pair of opposite words.

1. Arf/Earn

2. Girth/Felt

3. Thorn/Shout

4. Indies/Tedious

5. Stream/Taverns

Answers on page 318

HIDDEN QUOTATION

Cross out all words on the next page as instructed below. Then rearrange the remaining words (those that were not crossed out) to reveal a Buddhist proverb.

1. Cross out all brands of bicycles.

2. Cross out all precious metals.

3. Cross out all fish.

4. Cross out all four-syllable words.

5. Cross out all body parts.

6. Cross out all names of daily newspapers (cities not included).

long-term memory,
working memory,
attention to detail,
executive functioning

BEST	ANONYMOUS	CARP	LIP
A	UNIVERSAL	FOOL	REPLY
TOE	PLATINUM	SCHWINN	GOLD
IS	SILENCE	KNUCKLE	GLOBE
POST	COLUMBIA	HERALD	TIMES
TO	ELECTRIFY	PERCH	SILVER
THE	TRIBUNE	HUFFY	GUPPY

Quotation:

_____

_____

_____

Answers on page 318

It's All in the Name

long-term memory, multitasking, executive functioning

In this two-part game, you must first answer the clues, then put the answers in the correct order to reveal the name of a famous person. Here's a sample question: *The sound of a growl + Men's neckwear + The forest*. The answers are: *Grr + Tie + Woods*. Rearrange those answers and you get *Tie + Grr + Woods*.

1. Automobile + The fifth letter of the alphabet + North Korean dictator _____ Jong-un + A short quick run + Not out

2. A bowling alley + The fifth letter of the alphabet + Mr. Jagger of the Rolling Stones + To knock over a container of liquid

3. Automobile . . . with a Boston accent + Usual way to inflate a balloon + Tool used to break up ice + To use thread and a needle + Another word for Dad

Answers on page 318

ODD MAN OUT

In each list of items, all but one have something in common. Can you find the item that doesn't belong AND explain why it is the Odd Man Out?

1. Albany, Trenton, Santa Fe, Indianapolis

2. Period, Z, New Year's Eve, Amen, Hello

3. JPG, CIA, RAM, USB

4. Tin, Coffee, Telephone, Dixie

Answers on page 318

What's the Word?

Identify the missing letters that complete each row of words. For example, given the clues: _ _ _ **NERS, AL** _ _ _ **AC, HU** _ _ _ , _ _ _ **SION**, the correct answer is *MAN (Manners, Almanac, Human, Mansion). Note: All missing letters will form a three-letter word.*

JU _ _ _	INVO _ _ _	CHO _ _ _	L _ _ _ NSE
_ _ _ VE	S _ _ _ F	VI _ _ _	MAS _ _ _ A
_ _ _ LEX	P _ _ _ ER	CA _ _ _ UL	BA _ _ _ OOT
THR _ _ _	CH _ _ _ Y	M _ _ _ ION	P _ _ _ OW

Answers on page 318

Sentence Sleuth

A true Sentence Sleuth can find a type of BIRD hidden somewhere in each of these sentences. The correct answer could be spread over more than one word, and all punctuation, capital letters, etc., should be ignored.

1. When she saw both of her ex-husbands on the southbound train, Sarah awkwardly moved to a different car.

2. Catherine Whittington was ecstatic the day her oncologist said her cancer was in complete remission.

3. After he went to Hadrian's Wall, Owen decided to stay another week in northern England and Scotland.

Answers on page 318

Give Me a Word That . . .

You can make this into an especially challenging brain exercise if you answer each question completely within one minute.

1. Give me a word that . . . has five syllables.

_____

2. Give me two words that . . . end with the letter U.

_____

3. Give me four words that . . . contain a silent letter, such as *gnu*.

_____

_____

Answers on page 319

Common Bonds

long-term memory,
multitasking,
attention to detail

Find the common bond (or theme) among three very different pictures.

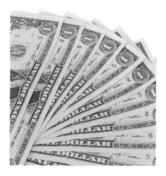

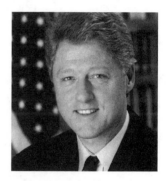

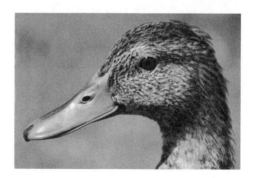

Answer on page 319

FIND THE THEME

The list below contains words that are all related to a theme.
Unscramble the words, then determine the theme.

ROOLSIE

_____

REDDOGS

_____

PARTIES

_____

DOXERS

_____

AEEKNSY

_____

THEME: _____

Answers on page 319

Addables

long-term memory, multitasking, attention to detail

Each clue in *Addables* contains a word with a success scale in parentheses. The goal is to make as many new words as possible in two minutes by adding one letter. With RUG, we found eight correct answers: **B**URG, **D**RUG, **F**RUG, GRU**B**, GURU, RUG**S**, RUN**G**, URG**E**. The success scale for RUG is 4 out of 8, which means that if you get four correct answers, you are doing well. Get more, and you're an Addable Expert! The second number indicates the total number of common English words we found for that clue.

1. WED   (5 out of 12)

2. COT   (4 out of 9)

3. INCH   (5 out of 8)

Answers on page 319

Do the Math!

Do you remember the arithmetic you learned in school? It's time to exercise your math smarts by solving this problem.

. . . .

On Monday, Farmer Joe got an order for fifteen dozen eggs. He has ninety chickens in the coop. Two thirds of his chickens lay one egg every day. The remaining one third have stopped laying (and are likely headed for the soup pot!).

How many days will it take for Farmer Joe to fill the order?

. . . .

Answer on page 319

Filled with Emotion

The clues in this game are all sayings, idioms, or titles that contain an "emotional" word that is missing. For example: _____ Baby (*Melancholy* Baby) or Fighting _____ (Fighting *mad*). Can you put back the missing emotions?

1. _____ sweet

2. _____ sack

3. _____ crime

4. _____ management

5. Bundle of _____

Answers on page 319

CHAPTER TWO

Low Intensity

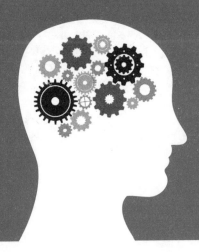

Need Directions?

We provide the name of some of the most famous streets, intersections, and highways in the world, both real and fictional. Can you identify the city, country, region—or story—where each is located?

1. The Beltway   _____

2. Abbey Road   _____

3. The Yellow Brick Road _____

4. The Grand Canal   _____

5. The Bowery   _____

6. Bourbon Street   _____

Answers on page 319

TRIMBLE

In this combination trivia game and word jumble, you must first answer the trivia questions (all related to car makes or models) and cross out the letters of each answer in the letter grid. Then rearrange the letters that have not been crossed out to reveal the Trimble answer.

1. This manufacturer introduced the Impala in 1957.

2. The official name of this car is the Volkswagen Type 1, but it's informally called Käfer in German and this in English.

3. The Charger and the Dart were popular cars made by this American manufacturer.

4. The country in which the Peugeot, Renault, and Citroën are made.

5. The logo of this British luxury company is also found on jet engines.

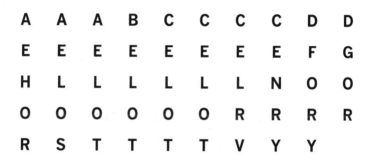

A	A	A	B	C	C	C	C	D	D
E	E	E	E	E	E	E	E	F	G
H	L	L	L	L	L	L	N	O	O
O	O	O	O	O	O	R	R	R	R
R	S	T	T	T	T	V	Y	Y	

Trimble Answer:

Word Jumble hint: The bestselling car model of all time.

Answers on page 319

Riddle Me This

working memory, attention to detail, executive functioning

Classic riddles like this one are easier to solve if you think outside the box.

....

Does England have a 4th of July?

....

Answer on page 320

Making Connections

Given six words in the grid, can you find the three pairs that belong together and explain why each is a pair?

ZIP	DASH
ESCORT	NADA
PINTO	COLON

In the sample above, one pair is *Escort* and *Pinto*, which are both Ford car models. Another pair is *Zip* and *Nada*, which both mean *nothing*. And *Dash* and *Colon* are both punctuation marks.

AREA	PIGGY
CREAM	RIVER
STRING	ZIP

Pair_____   Theme _____

Pair_____   Theme _____

Pair_____   Theme _____

Answers on page 320

TWO BY THREE

In this game, a three-letter word determines what your two answers can be. Let's take the word *WAR*, for example. If the first question is: *Name two authors for each letter*, the answers might be: **W**: *Thornton Wilder and H. G. Wells*, **A**: *Louisa May Alcott and Maya Angelou*, **R**: *Ayn Rand and Salman Rushdie*.

1. Name two types of flowers that start with each letter.

2. Name two dog breeds that start with each letter.

3. Name two diseases or conditions that start with each letter.

	Flowers	Dogs	Diseases
S			
A			
D			

Answers on page 320

SECRET Word

long-term memory, attention to detail, processing speed, executive functioning

How many four- or five-letter words can you find using the letters in the phrase below? The more words you find, the more likely you are to discover the secret word, which is generally a little harder to spot. (It's designated in the Solutions section.) To make this game a better brain exercise, try to find at least a dozen words in one minute.

QUILTING BEE

Answers on page 320

SAY WHAT?

Saul loves sayings and proverbs … but he can never remember them correctly. Can you fix his mistakes to reveal the correct saying? For example, Saul might say: "Humans who reside in clear, vitreous residences ought not to hurl small rocks." But the correct saying is: "People who live in glass houses should not throw stones."

1. "Excellent-quality boundary barriers create excellent-quality people who live very nearby."

   _____

2. "The discharge of atmospheric electricity at no time hits the identical location on two occasions."

   _____

3. "Create dried grass during the time that the star at the center of the Milky Way galaxy radiates."

   _____

4. "Spy the smallest coin, lift it, and for 24 hours you will experience serendipitous fortune."

   _____

5. "That which leaves in a circular fashion, returns in a circular fashion."

   _____

Answers on page 320

One-Minute Madness

How many FAMOUS PEOPLE WITH THE FIRST NAME GEORGE can you name in one minute?

_____

_____

_____

_____

_____

_____

_____

_____

_____

_____

_____

_____

_____

Answers on page 320

OTHER Words

long-term memory, attention to detail, executive functioning

Every word in this list is missing the letters **O-T-H-E-R**. Can you put those letters back (in any order) in the spaces below to reveal a common English word?

1. BA __ __ __ __ B __

2. __ A __ __ __ W __ RM

3. __ RC __ __ S __ __ A

4. T __ __ __ M __ S __ AT

5. G __ __ S __ WRIT __ __

6. BUT __ __ __ SC __ TC __

Answers on page 321

WORD TOWER

Build a tower of words that begins with the letters RE by increasing the number of letters in each consecutive word by one (example for the letters NO: NOT, NOON, NORTH, and so on). You cannot just add an S to a word already used, and no proper nouns are allowed. If you come up with words longer than eight letters, you're a Word Tower pro! *This game is a better brain booster if you put a one- or two-minute time limit on it.*

1. RE

2. RE __

3. RE __ __

4. RE __ __ __

5. RE __ __ __ __

6. RE __ __ __ __ __

7. RE __ __ __ __ __ __

8. RE __ __ __ __ __ __ __

Answers on page 321

Wacky Wordy

The arrangement of the letters in the frame is a clue to the answer. For example, if the word *school* were placed high up in the frame, the answer would be *high school*. Or if the phrase *easy pieces* occurred five times in the frame, the answer would be *five easy pieces*.

STA4NCE

Answer on page 321

People Rebus

Each picture rebus below represents the name of a famous person. Pay close attention to the plus and minus signs to know which sound to add or remove.

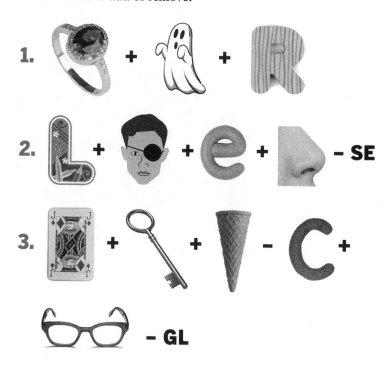

1. [ring] + [ghost] + [R]

2. [L] + [man with eye patch] + [e] + [nose] − SE

3. [Jack playing card] + [key] + [ice cream cone] − C + [glasses] − GL

Answers on page 321

What's the Word?

Identify the missing letters that complete each row of words. For example, given the clues: ___**NERS**, **AL**___**AC**, **HU**___, ___**SION**, the correct answer is *MAN (Manners, Almanac, Human, Mansion)*. *Note: All missing letters will form a three-letter word.*

PRO _ _ _	_ _ _ NESS	OUT _ _ _	GRAF _ _ _ I
_ _ _ EL	F _ _ _	_ _ _ DOG	COL _ _ _ SE
T _ _ _	_ _ _ ATE	P _ _ _ ECT	P _ _ _ EIN
_ _ _ SE	OP _ _ _	CAM _ _ _	C _ _ _ MICS

Answers on page 321

ODD MAN OUT

long-term memory,
working memory,
executive functioning

In each list of items, all but one have something in common. Can you find the item that doesn't belong AND explain why it is the Odd Man Out?

1. Rule, Retriever, Girls, Pencil

2. Chocolate, Casino, Potato, Guitar

3. Glory, Testament, Amendment, Age

4. Cotton, Horse, Saddle, Tap

Answers on page 321

Syllability

The answers to the questions below are made up only of syllables found in the grid. Cross out the syllables as you use them. The number in parentheses indicates the number of syllables in the answer.

1. A prison for people convicted of serious crimes (5)

_____

2. The outside boundary of a circle (4)

_____

3. DDT or Raid (4)

_____

4. Nil, zero (2)

_____

5. College commencement (4)

_____

long-term memory,
multitasking,
attention to detail,
executive functioning

6. Having no special or distinctive features, standard, typical (4)

_____

7. The totality of words known to a person (5)

_____

A	CAB	CIDE	CIR
CUM	DI	ENCE	FER
GRAD	I	IN	ING
LAR	NAR	NOTH	OR
PEN	RY	SEC	TEN
TI	TIA	TION	U
U	VO	Y	Y

Answers on page 321

OPPOSITES

ATTRACT

Rearrange the letters of each word provided to reveal a pair of opposite words.

1. Layer/Tale _____ _____

2. Slot/Fondu _____ _____

3. Niner/Route _____ _____

4. Cleric/Lien _____ _____

5. Owlets/Eighths _____ _____

Answers on page 321

Four Tricky Tongue Twisters!

Repeat each tongue twister three times quickly and out loud, without making a mistake.

Crash quiche course

Preshrunk silk shirts

Red Buick, blue Buick

Ted said Ed edited it

Change
a Letter

Change the three given words into new words by replacing one letter—without rearranging any of the existing letters. For example: PLAY, SNAIL, WAIST can be changed to PRAY, SNARL, WRIST. You can change any one of the existing letters, but you must use the same replacement letter for all three words.

1. Blown, Aloud, Soup   _____ _____ _____

2. Iron, Polite, Spatter   _____ _____ _____

3. Timer, Loiter, Pint   _____ _____ _____

4. Spa, Mouth, Math   _____ _____ _____

Answers on page 322

EIGHTS & Fours

Can you make one eight-letter word and two four-letter words from the scrambled letters below?

1.

D M P P R A E E

_ _ _ _ _ _ _ _

_ _ _ _

_ _ _ _

2.

E E U P R R S S

_ _ _ _ _ _ _ _

_ _ _ _

_ _ _ _

Answers on page 322

HIDDEN QUOTATION

Cross out all words on the next page as instructed below. Then rearrange the remaining words (those that were not crossed out) to reveal a quotation from humorist Will Rogers.

1. Cross out all diseases and conditions.

2. Cross out all synonyms for *smart*.

3. Cross out all rodents.

4. Cross out all traffic signs.

5. Cross out all prepositions.

6. Cross out all gemstones.

long-term memory,
working memory,
attention to detail,
executive functioning

ACROSS	YIELD	PAY	PORCUPINE
ASTHMA	NEAR	A	SHREWD
ONE WAY	UPON	RAT	COLD
OPAL	MAKE	STOP	BECOME
MERGE	GARNET	IN	TOPAZ
SQUIRREL	CRIME	FLU	INTO
LAWYER	STROKE	WISE	HAMSTER

Quotation:

_____

_____

_____

Answers on page 322

Fill In the Letters

Fill in the blank spaces with letters to make common English words. (No proper nouns are allowed.) For example, the clue __ **a t** yields twelve answers: *Bat, Cat, Eat, Fat, Hat, Mat, Oat, Pat, Rat, Sat, Tat, Vat. Note: The number in parentheses indicates how many common English words we found.* For a better cognitive workout, put a one-minute timer on each puzzle below.

1. _ **UT** _   (21)

2. _ _ **KER**   (14)

Answers on page 322

Give Me a Word That . . .

You can make this into an especially challenging brain exercise if you answer each question completely within one minute.

1. Give me eight words that . . . rhyme with *sleep*.

2. Give me four words that . . . mean *angry*.

3. Give me three words that . . . contain the letter J, but NOT in the first position.

Answers on page 322

Griddle

Find as many words with four or more connected letters as you can in two minutes. The letters must touch either vertically, horizontally, or diagonally. You cannot skip or jump across letters and you cannot use the same letter twice in one word. For example, to make the word *loyal*, you must have two Ls in the grid. Proper nouns are not allowed.

R	A	N	T
E	I	F	E
N	F	O	F
T	N	U	L

working memory,
multitasking,
attention to detail,
processing speed

_____   _____   _____

_____   _____   _____

_____   _____   _____

_____   _____   _____

_____   _____   _____

_____   _____   _____

_____   _____   _____

_____   _____   _____

_____   _____   _____

_____   _____   _____

_____   _____   _____

_____   _____   _____

_____   _____   _____

_____   _____   _____

Answers on page 322

Order, Please!

long-term memory,
working memory,
multitasking,
executive functioning

Given a list of three or four items, your job is to rearrange them in the order called for in the question.

1. Put these units of measurement in order by size, starting with the largest:

_____ 1 liter

_____ 1 gallon

_____ 3 cups

2. Put these women in order by date of birth, starting with the oldest:

_____ Elizabeth Warren

_____ Angela Merkel

_____ Hillary Clinton

Answers on page 322

Run the Alphabet

long-term memory, working memory, processing speed

From *Albania* to *Zimbabwe*, we're looking for the name of a COUNTRY for each letter of the alphabet. This game is a better brain booster if you put a two- or three-minute timer on it.

A_____ H_____ O_____ V_____

B_____ I_____ P_____ W *(none)*

C_____ J_____ Q_____ X *(none)*

D_____ K_____ R_____ Y_____

E_____ L_____ S_____ Z_____

F_____ M_____ T_____

G_____ N_____ U_____

Answers on page 323

DOUBLE TROUBLE

Given a list of words such as *knuckle*, *moth*, and *basket*, can you find the one word that follows each of them to make a compound word or two-word phrase? For the example words above, the correct answer is *ball* (*knuckleball*, *mothball*, and *basketball*). *Note: The first letter of each answer is provided in a hint below ... but try not to use it unless you're really stuck!*

1. Funeral, Broken, Motor

2. Direct, Fan, Voice

3. Duty, Fancy, Fat

4. Sand, Death, Mouse

(Hints: 1-H, 2-M, 3-F, 4-T)

Answers on page 323

What's the Word?

Identify the missing letters that complete each row of words. For example, given the clues: _ _ _ **NERS, AL**_ _ _ **AC, HU**_ _ _, _ _ _ **SION**, the correct answer is *MAN* (*Manners, Almanac, Human, Mansion*). *Note: All missing letters will form a three-letter word.*

_ _ _ ION	C _ _ _ US	F _ _ _ ORY	COMP _ _ _
_ _ _ B	CI _ _ _	SU _ _ _	_ _ _ DEN
S _ _ _ E	C _ _ _ BER	_ _ _ LET	_ _ _ STER
CO _ _ _	_ _ _ RO	_ _ _ HOD	DIA _ _ _ ER

Answers on page 323

Pictures & Letters

By combining one picture and one letter name (Cee, Bee, El, Pea, En, and Eye), can you come up with six new words?

C	B	L
P	N	I

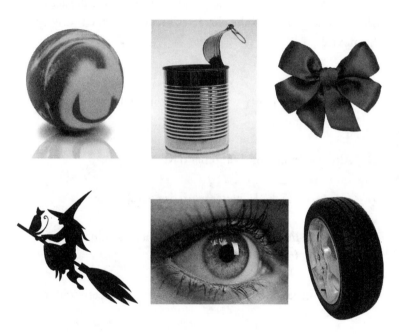

Answers on page 323

Memorable
Movie Lines

These movie lines are well known; but can you name the actor who spoke the line, OR the character's name, OR the title of the movie?

1. "Of all the gin joints in all the towns in all the world, she walks into mine."

2. "After all, tomorrow is another day!"

3. "Greed, for lack of a better word, is good."

4. "Listen to me, mister. You're my knight in shining armor. Don't you forget it."

5. "It's a Sicilian message. It means Luca Brasi sleeps with the fishes."

Answers on page 323

Counting Syllables

long-term memory, multitasking, processing speed, executive functioning

Come up with the answers to these questions, syllable by syllable. Put a one-minute timer on each question and you'll get a better brain workout.

1. Name four types of pasta with four-syllable names.

2. Name three items of furniture with two-syllable names.

3. Name one movie with a one-syllable title.

4. Name the only US state with a one-syllable name.

Answers on page 323

One-Minute Madness

long-term memory,
working memory,
processing speed

How many NETWORK AND CABLE TELEVISION
OUTLETS can you name in one minute? (If you come up with
more than a dozen, you're a TV expert!)

_____

_____

_____

_____

_____

_____

_____

_____

_____

_____

_____

Answers on page 324

Finish
the Proverb

Given just the last two words of a well-known proverb or saying, can you fill in the rest?

1. _____ the crime.

2. _____ do today.

3. _____ are free.

4. _____ good thing.

Answers on page 324

Picture Connections

Find the three groups of three related pictures and explain why they are connected. For example, if three of the nine pictures were *Johnny Carson*, *Jay Leno*, and *Jimmy Fallon*, they would be connected as *Tonight Show hosts*.

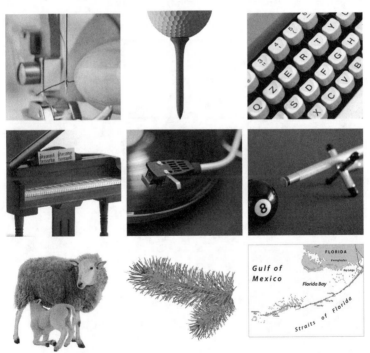

Answers on page 324

Presidential
Quotations

long-term memory,
working memory,
executive functioning

Can you match the quote with the US president who said it?

1. "There is nothing wrong in America that can't be fixed with what is right in America."

2. "If government is to serve any purpose, it is to do for others what they are unable to do for themselves."

3. "Change will not come if we wait for some other person, or if we wait for some other time. We are the ones we've been waiting for. We are the change that we seek."

4. "You want a friend in Washington? Get a dog."

a. Barack Obama

b. Harry Truman

c. Lyndon Johnson

d. Bill Clinton

Answers on page 324

HAPPY ENDINGS

Can you come up with the missing letters that complete each set of words? Here's an example:

| CA____ | SWE____ | OBSE____ | CONSE____ |

The correct answer is **RVE (CARVE, SWERVE, OBSERVE, CONSERVE)**.

1	VO____	FIS____	RAS____	LOGI____
2	ST____	LOV____	PORT____	IRRIT____
3	SW____	BAB____	BUFF____	MACAR____
4	NA____	FES____	CREA____	FUGI____

Answers on page 324

It's All in the Name

long-term memory, multitasking, executive functioning

In this two-part game, you must first answer the clues, then put the answers in the correct order to reveal the name of a famous person. Here's a sample question: *The sound of a growl + Men's neckwear + The forest*. The answers are: *Grr + Tie + Woods*. Rearrange those answers and you get *Tie + Grr + Woods*.

1. To break in and steal things + A sticky or slimy substance + To cause physical injury or pain to someone + Hawaiian flower necklace

2. A precious gem + The fourth letter of the alphabet + The fifth letter of the alphabet + The little orphan of comic strip fame + Discourteous, bad-mannered

3. An injury caused by high heat or fire + The opposite of even + Point where the legs meet the pelvis + Memo word that means *in the matter of*

Answers on page 325

A Potpourri of Nicknames

Can you identify these people, places, and things by their nicknames?

1. The Tube _____

2. Soup Strainer _____

3. Shrub _____

4. Old Glory _____

5. Lady Lindy _____

Answers on page 325

Join 'Em

working memory,
multitasking,
attention to detail,
executive functioning

Join together any two words from the columns on the left below, putting an R in the middle, to create one longer word. For example: *PA* plus *ROT* with an *R* in the middle is *PARROT*. While there might be alternatives, only one way works for all the words. *Note: The shorter words can come from the same column or both columns.*

SHORT WORDS		LONGER WORDS
ABLE	AGE	1 _____ **R** _____
ALLY	ANT	2 _____ **R** _____
ATE	CHANT	3 _____ **R** _____
GENE	ME	4 _____ **R** _____
MEMO	OUT	5 _____ **R** _____
PI	WAR	6 _____ **R** _____

Answers on page 325

Sentence Sleuth

long-term memory, multitasking, attention to detail, executive functioning

A true Sentence Sleuth can find the name of a DANCE (of any type) hidden somewhere in each of these sentences. The correct answer could be spread over more than one word, and all punctuation, capital letters, etc., should be ignored.

1. "You're not old," said Charles to Nana Mary, "you are just experienced."

2. I found out that Felicity's husband is co-editor of *The Oxford American Dictionary*.

3. Tipper Gore once said that "As Time Goes By" is Al's all-time favorite song.

Answers on page 325

OPPOSITES
ATTRACT

Rearrange the letters of each word provided to reveal a pair of opposite words.

1. Grown/Girth　　　_____　_____

2. Rove/Nuder　　　_____　_____

3. Tarts/Post　　　_____　_____

4. Cheat/Renal　　　_____　_____

5. Coles/Pone　　　_____　_____

Answers on page 325

DOWN TO THE WIRE

long-term memory,
working memory,
processing speed

Put back the word or words that complete each expression.
This is a better brain booster if you complete all the questions in one minute.

1. _____ to the plate

2. _____ to the chase

3. _____ to the teeth

4. _____ to the Galaxy

5. _____ to the slaughter

Answers on page 325

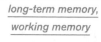
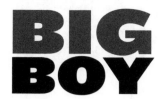

The answer to each clue is a word, name, phrase, or saying that contains the word BIG.

1. IBM's nickname

_____

2. The leading explanation for how the universe began from small dense matter and expanded outward

_____

3. A group of seven stars in the constellation Ursa Major

_____

4. More pressing concerns, more important things to do

_____

5. Proverb that Theodore Roosevelt used to describe his foreign policy

_____

Answers on page 325

Stinky Pinky

Each Stinky Pinky answer contains two words that rhyme. Can you figure out what the answer is from an offbeat definition? For example, the answer to the clue *Mrs. Onassis's tan pants* is *Jackie's khakis*.

1. Homily in Berlin

2. Soft French cheese at no cost

3. In-shape London resident

4. Eating utensil made from a dried plum

5. The funniest joke

Answers on page 325

FORE
Words

long-term memory,
attention to detail,
executive functioning

Every word in this list is missing the letters **F-O-R-E**. Can you put those letters back (in any order) in the spaces below to reveal a common English word?

1. __ __ **F** __ __

2. **B** __ **N** __ **I** __ __

3. __ __ __ __ **IGN**

4. **BA** __ __ __ **O** __ **T**

5. **IN** __ __ **RI** __ __

6. **B** __ **Y** __ __ **I** __ **ND**

Answers on page 325

CHAPTER THREE

Get in Gear

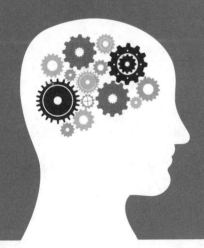

Movie
Questions

In what movie would you hear these famous questions?

1. "Hey Dad, you wanna have a catch?"

2. "You gotta ask yourself one question: 'Do I feel lucky?' Well, do ya, punk?"

3. "You talking to me?"

4. "Who ya gonna call?"

5. "You want answers?"
"I want the truth!"
"You can't handle the truth!"

Answers on page 326

Riddle Me This

Classic riddles like this one are easier to solve if you think outside the box.

....

How can a woman living in Canada legally marry three men without ever getting a divorce, being widowed, or becoming legally separated?

....

Answer on page 326

One-Minute Madness

How many words that mean A LIE or TO LIE can you come up with in one minute?

_____

_____

_____

_____

_____

_____

_____

_____

_____

_____

_____

_____

Answers on page 326

Addables

Each clue in *Addables* contains a word with a success scale in parentheses. The goal is to make as many new words as possible in two minutes by adding one letter and scrambling all the letters. With RUG, we found eight correct answers: **B**RUG, **D**RUG, **F**RUG, GRU**B**, GUR**U**, RUG**S**, RU**N**G, UR**G**E. The success scale for RUG is 4 out of 8, which means that if you get four correct answers, you are doing well. Get more, and you're an Addable Expert! The second number indicates the total number of common English words we found for that clue.

1. NAP   (6 out of 11)

2. DIG   (3 out of 5)

3. FED   (4 out of 8)

Answers on page 326

Mathematically
Speaking

Although the questions in this quiz have little or nothing to do with math, all of the answers do. For example, the answer to the clue *An Egyptian burial tomb* is *pyramid* (which, mathematically speaking, is a geometric shape).

1. You don't want to see a long one when you go to renew your driver's license.

2. The headquarters building of the US military.

3. A carpentry tool used to smooth a wooden surface.

4. A substitute for mother's milk.

5. This is one way to park a car.

Answers on page 326

Is or Isn't?

long-term memory, working memory, executive functioning

In this game, you have to find the one item in each list that is—or isn't—what we say it is . . . or isn't.

1. Which actor is . . . in the 1991 film *The Silence of the Lambs*?
   a. Ben Kingsley
   b. Michael Caine
   c. Anthony Hopkins
   d. Julia Roberts

2. Which one isn't . . . an Ivy League college?
   a. Rutgers University
   b. Brown University
   c. Dartmouth College
   d. Cornell University

3. Which animal is . . . a marsupial?
   a. Squirrel
   b. Koala
   c. Beaver
   d. Porcupine

4. Which city isn't . . . on a seacoast?
   a. Washington, DC
   b. New Orleans, LA
   c. Portland, ME
   d. Vancouver, BC, Canada

Answers on page 326

Filled
with Emotion

long-term memory, working memory

The clues in this game are all sayings, idioms, or titles that contain an "emotional" word that is missing. For example:
_____ Baby (*Melancholy* Baby) or Fighting _____ (Fighting *mad*). Can you put back the missing emotions?

1. _____ Bull

2. The Sound and the _____

3. _____ of Flying

4. Swallow your _____

5. _____ hour

Answers on page 326

Griddle

Find as many words with four or more connected letters as you can in two minutes. The letters must touch either vertically, horizontally, or diagonally. You cannot skip or jump across letters, and you cannot use the same letter twice in one word. For example, to make the word *loyal*, you must have two Ls in the grid. Proper nouns are not allowed.

A	N	D	I
R	E	F	T
H	C	E	F
E	L	E	R

_____ _____ _____

_____ _____ _____

_____ _____ _____

_____ _____ _____

_____ _____ _____

_____ _____ _____

_____ _____ _____

_____ _____ _____

_____ _____ _____

_____ _____ _____

_____ _____ _____

_____ _____ _____

_____ _____ _____

_____ _____ _____

_____ _____ _____

Answers on page 326

EIGHTS
& Fours

Can you make one eight-letter word and two four-letter words from the scrambled letters below?

1. IOHPRSSW

— — — — — — — —

— — — —

— — — —

2. AEPRSTTY

— — — — — — — —

— — — —

— — — —

Answers on page 327

JiNGLES & SLOGANS

Finish the jingle or advertising slogan, and then name the product (unless it's already named in the clue or answer).

1. "You got chocolate in _____."

   _____

2. "It takes a tough man _____."

   _____

3. "For everything else, there's _____."

   _____

4. "Where's the _____?"

   _____

5. "We're looking for a few _____."

   _____

Answers on page 327

Wacky Wordy

The arrangement of the letters in the frame is a clue to the answer. For example, if the word *school* were placed high up in the frame, the answer would be *high school*. Or if the phrase *easy pieces* occurred five times in the frame, the answer would be *five easy pieces*.

OTHER FOOT

Answer on page 327

Homographs

long-term memory, attention to detail, executive functioning

Homographs are a type of homonym in which two or more words are spelled the same but have different meanings. Given two definitions, can you identify the homograph?

1. A brand of wristwatch and the legal resident of a country

2. The astrological birth sign for June and July and a large group of diseases involving abnormal cell growth

3. Generic term for an item of clothing worn on the upper part of the human body and a child's toy

4. Experience the hallucinogenic effect of LSD and stumble over an object

5. A small fruit and a bird

Answers on page 327

GET IN GEAR   111

The Name of the Game

Can you fill in the missing first name or surname from each saying or idiom?

1. The real _____

2. _____ horse

3. _____ club

4. _____ on the spot

5. Smart _____

Answers on page 327

Making Connections

Given six words in the grid, can you find the three pairs that belong together and explain why each is a pair?

ZIP	DASH
ESCORT	NADA
COLON	PINTO

In the sample above, one pair is *Escort* and *Pinto*, which are both Ford car models. Another pair is *Zip* and *Nada*, which both mean *nothing*. And *Dash* and *Colon* are both punctuation marks.

KEY	INCOME
CHECK	NAPKIN
PROPERTY	TRAMPOLINE

Pair_____   Theme _____

Pair_____   Theme _____

Pair_____   Theme _____

Answers on page 327

SECRET
Word

long-term memory,
attention to detail,
processing speed,
executive functioning

How many four- or five-letter words can you find using the letters in the phrase below? The more words you find, the more likely you are to discover the secret word, which is generally a little harder to spot. (It's designated in the Solutions section.) To make this game a better brain exercise, try to find at least a dozen words in one minute.

TOOTHPASTE

Answers on page 327

SAY WHAT?

Saul loves sayings and proverbs . . . but he can never remember them correctly. Can you fix his mistakes to reveal the correct saying? For example, Saul might say: "Humans who reside in clear, vitreous residences ought not to hurl small rocks." But the correct saying is: "People who live in glass houses should not throw stones."

1. "The rotating circle with the high-pitched sound receives the lubricant."

_____

_____

2. "Every beneficial entity has to reach a conclusion."

_____

_____

3. "One image has the value of 10 times 100 spoken units of language."

_____

_____

4. "The passage of minutes and hours equals bills and coins."

_____

_____

5. "Red body fluid is more viscous than H_2O."

_____

_____

Answers on page 328

Word Rebus

Each picture rebus represents a word. Pay close attention to the plus and minus signs to know which sound to add or remove.

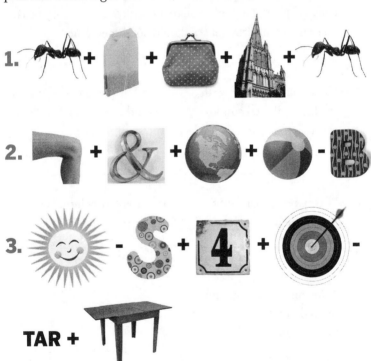

1.

2.

3.

TAR +

Answers on page 328

Your Highness

The answer to each clue is a name, title, or phrase, that contains the royal title KING or QUEEN.

1. Tennis great

_____

2. A brand of flour

_____

3. 1951 movie starring Humphrey Bogart and Katharine Hepburn

_____

4. The second-largest state in Australia

_____

5. Moniker for Benny Goodman

_____

Answers on page 328

Scrambled States

Unscramble the letters in these unusual phrases to reveal the name of a US state. You can make this a better brain workout if you can unscramble all the state names in two minutes!

1. COOL ROAD _____

2. LOOK A HAM _____

3. NOT A MAN _____

4. IN NAVY PLANES _____

5. COAL TRAIN HORN _____

Answers on page 328

Endings & Beginnings

In this game, we provide the first half of one compound word or two-word phrase and the second half of another. Can you come up with the one word that completes both? *Note: The first letter of each answer is provided in a hint below . . . but try not to use it unless you're really stuck!*

1. Like   _____   Crack

2. Care   _____   Way

3. Fire   _____   Chair

4. Clock _____   Active

5. Bitter _____   Heart

Give Me a Word That . . .

working memory, multitasking, attention to detail, processing speed

You can make this into an especially challenging brain exercise if you answer each question completely within one minute.

1. Give me three words that . . . have more than eight letters.

_____

2. Give me twelve words that . . . have only two letters.

_____

3. Give me two words that . . . are compound words (two words that together form a new word, such as *butterfly* or *peppermint*).

_____

Answers on page 328

What's the Word?

working memory, attention to detail, executive functioning

Identify the missing letters that complete each row of words. For example, given the clues: _ _ _ **NERS**, **AL**_ _ _ **AC**, **HU**_ _ _, _ _ _ **SION**, the correct answer is *MAN* (*Manners, Almanac, Human, Mansion*). *Note: All missing letters will form a three-letter word.*

_ _ _ ATE	ABAN _ _ _	_ _ _ KEY	TEN _ _ _
_ _ _ SIDE	M _ _ _ H	B _ _ _ IQUE	DEV _ _ _
D _ _ _ DLE	_ _ _ DOW	SNO _ _ _ G	T _ _ _ KLE
AF _ _ _ D	COM _ _ _ T	_ _ _ BID	BE _ _ _ E

Answers on page 329

Run the Alphabet

long-term memory, working memory, processing speed

From *Applebee's* to *Zappos*, we're looking for the name of a COMPANY (of any type) for each letter of the alphabet. This game is a better brain booster if you put a two- or three-minute timer on it.

A_____   H_____   O_____   V_____

B_____   I_____   P_____   W_____

C_____   J_____   Q_____   X_____

D_____   K_____   R_____   Y_____

E_____   L_____   S_____   Z_____

F_____   M_____   T_____

G_____   N_____   U_____

Answers on page 329

WORD TOWER

long-term memory,
processing speed,
executive functioning

Build a tower of words that begins with the letters TO by increasing the number of letters in each consecutive word by one (example for the letters NO: NOT, NOON, NORTH, and so on). You cannot just add an S to a word already used, and no proper nouns are allowed. If you come up with words longer than eight letters, you're a Word Tower pro! *This game is a better brain booster if you put a one- or two-minute time limit on it.*

1. TO

2. TO __

3. TO __ __

4. TO __ __ __

5. TO __ __ __ __

6. TO __ __ __ __ __

7. TO __ __ __ __ __ __

8. TO __ __ __ __ __ __ __

Answers on page 329

ODD MAN OUT

long-term memory, working memory, executive functioning

In each list of items, all but one have something in common. Can you find the item that doesn't belong AND explain why it is the Odd Man Out?

1. Eyes, Arms, Nose, Knees

2. Dean, North, Hunt, Liddy

3. Britain, Dane, Scott, Turk

4. *Chariots of Fire, Angela's Ashes, Bloody Sunday, In the Name of the Father*

Answers on page 329

Change a Letter

Change the three given words into new words by replacing one letter—without rearranging any of the existing letters. For example: PLAY, SNAIL, WAIST can be changed to PRAY, SNARL, WRIST. You can change any one of the existing letters, but you must use the same replacement letter for all three words.

1. Toe, Binge, Prone _____ _____ _____

2. Ilk, Patio, Player _____ _____ _____

3. Knee, Eager, Never _____ _____ _____

4. Chatter, Slow, Ballet _____ _____ _____

Answers on page 329

Letter Play

long-term memory, multitasking, attention to detail

The goal of this game is to come up with the Letter Play Word at the bottom of the page. To do that, you must 1) finish each word in the list with the correct letter, chosen from the options in parentheses. Then 2) place that letter in the blank space of the Letter Play Word that corresponds with its clue number.

1. COU__T   (N, R)

2. DAN__ER   (C, G)

3. GR__NT   (A, U)

4. PA__TY   (T, R)

5. T__CK   (A, I)

6. CR__ED   (E, I)

7. LAM__   (B, P)

___ ___ ___ ___ ___ ___ ___
7 3 4 2 5 6 1

Answers on page 329

OPPOSITES

multitasking, executive functioning

ATTRACT

Rearrange the letters of each word provided to reveal a pair of opposite words.

1. Now/Slot _____ _____

2. Nope/Thus _____ _____

3. Veils/Side _____ _____

4. Vase/Pends _____ _____

5. Bets/Trows _____ _____

Answers on page 330

HIDDEN QUOTATION

Cross out all words on the next page as instructed below. Then rearrange the remaining words (those that were not crossed out) to reveal a quotation from Ralph Waldo Emerson.

1. Cross out all words that begin with a vowel (not including Y).

2. Cross out all US presidents' last names.

3. Cross out all words that form different words reading backward and forward (such as *wolf/flow*).

4. Cross out all two-syllable words that have double letters.

5. Cross out all three-syllable words with five letters.

6. Cross out all names of planets.

long-term memory,
working memory,
attention to detail,
executive functioning

WILL	BUTTER	TO	NIP
EAT	BECOME	VENUS	GIRAFFE
STOP	MANIA	UNDER	PERSON
DECIDE	ARSON	RADIO	DEVIL
MARS	JUPITER	MAY	YOU
INK	BE	VIDEO	YOU
THE	FLUFFY	BUSH	OVER

Quotation:

_____

_____

_____

Answers on page 330

Do the Math!

Do you remember the arithmetic you learned in school? It's time to exercise your math smarts by solving this problem.

....

When Amy was making a scarf, she kept a diary of each time she picked up and put down her knitting needles. From the following schedule, can you calculate how long it took her to make the scarf?

8:05 a.m. to 9:22 a.m.
11:51 a.m. to 1:37 p.m.
7:45 p.m. to 10:52 p.m.

....

Answer on page 330

Four Tricky Tongue Twisters!

Repeat each tongue twister three times quickly and out loud, without making a mistake.

Freshly fried flying fish

So this is the sushi chef

Seventy-seven benevolent elephants

Are our oars oak?

FOOL
Words

Every word in this list is missing the letters F-O-O-L. Can you put those letters back (in any order) in the spaces below to reveal a common English word?

1. __ __ L __ __ W

2. __ __ R __ __ RN

3. SP __ __ N __ U __

4. __ __ XH __ __ E

5. __ A __ SEH __ __ D

6. CHI __ DPR __ __ __

Answers on page 330

Is or Isn't?

In this game, you have to find the one item in each list that is—or isn't—what we say it is . . . or isn't.

1. Which of the following isn't . . . a Native American tribe?
   a. Shoshone
   b. Nez Perce
   c. Mezquita
   d. Clackamas

2. Which of the following isn't . . . a cheese?
   a. Burrata
   b. Cimarron
   c. Halloumi
   d. Fontina

3. Which of the following isn't . . . a mammal?
   a. Dolphin
   b. Rat
   c. Moose
   d. Shark

4. Which of the following is . . . a geometrical shape?
   a. Hexapod
   b. Trilogy
   c. Pentagon
   d. Octavo

Answers on page 330

One-Minute Madness

How many US CITIES THAT BEGIN WITH SAN OR SANTA can you name in one minute?

_____

_____

_____

_____

_____

_____

_____

_____

_____

_____

_____

Answers on page 330

Animal
Watching

These are not animals we see every day. Can you identify them?

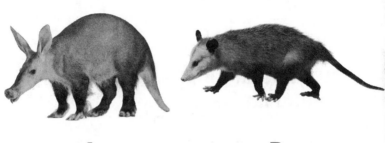

A.

B.

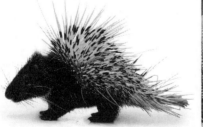

C.

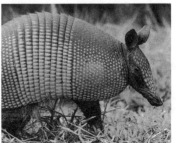

D.

Answers on page 330

A Pair of Riddles

Classic riddles like these are easier to solve if you think outside the box.

....

1. **What jumps higher than a building?**

2. **What kind of tree do you carry in your hand?**

....

Answers on page 330

DOUBLE TROUBLE

Given a list of words such as *knuckle*, *moth*, and *basket*, can you find the one word that follows each of them to make a compound word or two-word phrase? For the example words above, the correct answer is *ball* (*knuckleball*, *mothball*, and *basketball*). *Note: The first letter of each answer is provided in a hint below . . . but try not to use it unless you're really stuck!*

1. Wiggle, Elbow, Hotel

_____

2. Air, Hip, Pick

_____

3. Bull, Pillow, Dog

_____

4. Half, Sand, Silver

_____

(Hints: 1-R, 2-P, 3-F, 4-D)

Answers on page 330

Wacky Wordy

The arrangement of the letters in the frame is a clue to the answer. For example, if the word *school* were placed high up in the frame, the answer would be *high school*. Or if the phrase *easy pieces* occurred five times in the frame, the answer would be *five easy pieces*.

.That's

Answer on page 330

COLORFILL

Put back the missing color in each phrase, saying, or idiom.

1. _____ light district

2. _____ journalism

3. Talk a _____ streak

4. _____ heart

Answers on page 330

Picture Connections

Find the three groups of three related pictures and explain why they are connected. For example, if three of the nine pictures were *Johnny Carson*, *Jay Leno*, and *Jimmy Fallon*, they would be connected as *Tonight Show hosts*.

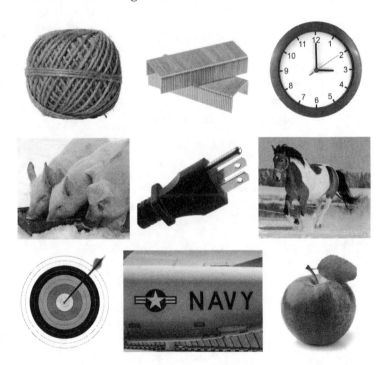

Answers on page 331

Counting Syllables

Come up with the answers to these questions, syllable by syllable. Put a one-minute timer on each question and you'll get a better brain workout.

1. Name four types of fabric/textiles with one-syllable names.

_____

2. Name four car companies with three-syllable names.

_____

3. Name ten animals (of any type) with one-syllable names.

_____

4. Identify six US cities with two-syllable names.

_____

Answers on page 331

Finish the Proverb

Given just the last two words of a well-known proverb or saying, can you fill in the rest?

1. _____ friend indeed.

2. _____ a rug.

3. _____ must fall.

4. _____ the dawn.

Answers on page 331

Sentence Sleuth

long-term memory,
multitasking,
attention to detail,
executive functioning

A true Sentence Sleuth can find the name of a FRUIT hidden somewhere in each of these sentences. The correct answer could be spread over more than one word, and all punctuation, capital letters, etc., should be ignored.

1. After a credible terrorist threat was made, the FBI decided to wiretap pledges at all Cal Tech fraternities.

2. When the steering broke on her mother-in-law's 1966 Mustang, Erin escaped with just a broken arm.

3. The nurse said that Dr. Bergman is available Mondays and Fridays in March.

Answers on page 331

Seeing ★ Stars ★

The answer to each clue is a title or phrase that contains the word STAR.

1. Texas's nickname

_____

2. Symbol of modern Judaism and the nation of Israel

_____

3. The US national anthem

_____

4. Hoagy Carmichael's 1927 song that begins: "Sometimes I wonder why I spend the lonely nights dreaming of a song . . ."

_____

5. Description of lovers, such as Romeo and Juliet, who are thwarted by bad luck

_____

Answers on page 331

Common Bonds

long-term memory,
multitasking,
attention to detail

Find the common bond (or theme) among three very different pictures.

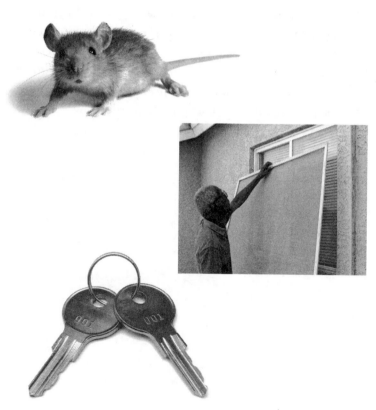

Answer on page 331

Fill In the Letters

Fill in the blank spaces with letters to make common English words. (No proper nouns are allowed.) For example, the clue __ **a t** yields twelve answers: *Bat, Cat, Eat, Fat, Hat, Mat, Oat, Pat, Rat, Sat, Tat, Vat. Note: The number in parentheses indicates how many common English words we found.* For a better cognitive workout, put a one-minute timer on each puzzle below.

1. _ _ **RD** _   (12)

2. _ **ID** _   (13)

Answers on page 331

Order, Please!

Given a list of three or four items, your job is to rearrange them in the order called for in the question.

1. Put this list of foods in order of their calorie count, starting with the least caloric:

_____One medium banana

_____One large hard-boiled egg

_____One cup of peas

2. Put these US states in order by landmass, starting with the largest:

_____Washington

_____New York

_____Nevada

Answers on page 332

CHAPTER FOUR

Dig
Deep!

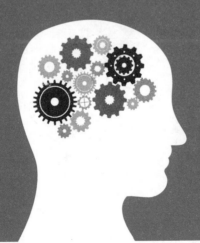

Stinky Pinky

Each Stinky Pinky answer contains two words that rhyme. Can you figure out what the answer is from an offbeat definition? For example, the answer to the clue *Mrs. Onassis's tan pants* is *Jackie's khakis.*

1. A feeble person from Athens

2. Prince Charles's mother after a bath

3. Lock openers made of gouda

4. A yellow fruit from the capital of Cuba

5. A traditional song about a bowl of greens and other raw vegetables

Answers on page 332

Addables

Each clue in *Addables* contains a word with a success scale in parentheses. The goal is to make as many new words as possible in two minutes by adding one letter and scrambling all the letters. With RUG, we found eight correct answers: **B**URG, **D**RUG, **F**RUG, GRU**B**, GUR**U**, RUG**S**, RUN**G**, **U**RG**E**. The success scale for RUG is 4 out of 8, which means that if you get four correct answers, you are doing well. Get more, and you're an Addable Expert! The second number indicates the total number of common English words we found for that clue.

1. BUST   (5 out of 10)

2. GRIN   (3 out of 9)

3. HERE   (3 out of 6)

Answers on page 332

SECRET
Word

long-term memory,
attention to detail,
processing speed,
executive functioning

How many four- or five-letter words can you find using the letters in the phrase below? The more words you find, the more likely you are to discover the secret word, which is generally a little harder to spot. (It's designated in the Solutions section.) To make this game a better brain exercise, try to find at least a dozen words in one minute.

> **FRIED FISH**

Answers on page 332

ACRONYM ALPHABET

What do these common acronyms stand for?

1. BMW _____

2. FCC _____

3. MASH _____

4. VCR _____

5. CPR _____

6. ROTC _____

Answers on page 332

People
Rebus

Each picture rebus below represents a famous person's name. Pay close attention to the plus and minus signs to know which sounds to add or remove.

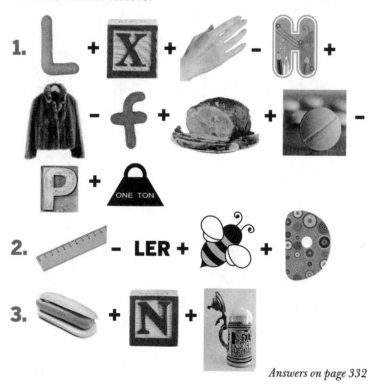

Answers on page 332

WORD TOWER

Build a tower of words that begins with the letters AL by increasing the number of letters in each consecutive word by one (example for the letters NO: NOT, NOON, NORTH, and so on). You cannot just add an S to a word already used, and no proper nouns are allowed. If you come up with words longer than eight letters, you're a Word Tower pro! *This game is a better brain booster if you put a one- or two-minute time limit on it.*

1. AL

2. AL __

3. AL __ __

4. AL __ __ __

5. AL __ __ __ __

6. AL __ __ __ __ __

7. AL __ __ __ __ __ __

8. AL __ __ __ __ __ __ __

Answers on page 333

EIGHTS & Fours

Can you make one eight-letter word and two four-letter words from the scrambled letters below?

1.

A E E O D L M N

— — — — — — — —

— — — —

— — — —

2.

A O F L M P R T

— — — — — — — —

— — — —

— — — —

Answers on page 333

Give Me a Word That . . .

You can make this into an especially challenging brain exercise if you answer each question completely within one minute.

1. Give me six words with four or more letters that . . . contain double letters, such as *doodle* or *apple*.

2. Give me six words with four or more letters that . . . end in B.

3. Give me the one word that . . . ends the US Pledge of Allegiance.

Answers on page 333

One-Minute Madness

long-term memory,
working memory,
processing speed

In a baseball game there can be as many as nineteen people (players, coaches, and officiators) on the playing field at one time (not counting base runners). How many of these nineteen BASEBALL POSITIONS can you name in one minute?

_____

_____

_____

_____

_____

_____

_____

_____

_____

_____

Answers on page 333

TWO BY THREE

In this game, a three-letter word determines what your two answers can be. Let's take the word *WAD*, for example. If the first question is: *Name two authors for each letter*, the answers might be: **W**: *Thornton Wilder and H. G. Wells*, **A**: *Louisa May Alcott and Maya Angelou*, **D**: *Charles Dickens and Joan Didion*.

1. Name two types of insects that start with each letter.

2. Come up with two six-letter words that start with each letter.

3. Name two US cities that start with each letter.

	Insects	6-Letter Words	US Cities
C			
A			
B			

Answers on page 333

SAY WHAT?

Saul loves sayings and proverbs ... but he can never remember them correctly. Can you fix his mistakes to reveal the correct saying? For example, Saul might say: "Humans who reside in clear, vitreous residences ought not to hurl small rocks." But the correct saying is: "People who live in glass houses should not throw stones."

1. "Not within one's visual field, not within one's brain."

_____

2. "Not a thing exists as a gratis midday repast."

_____

3. "If you desire an indeterminate thing accomplished correctly, perform it on your own."

_____

4. "Converse for the duration it takes for your mug to become a shade of azure."

_____

5. "That's the manner in which the baked good falls into pieces."

_____

Answers on page 333

Syllability

The answers to the questions below are made up only of syllables found in the grid. Cross out the syllables as you use them. The number in parentheses indicates the number of syllables in the answer.

1. The first book of the Bible (3)

_____

2. The "vast wasteland," according to Newton Minow (4)

_____

3. Letter container (3)

_____

4. Key ingredient in guacamole (4)

_____

5. Toll House or Newton (2)

_____

long-term memory,
multitasking,
attention to detail,
executive functioning

6. Individually owned apartment (5)

_____

7. Prehistoric giants (3)

_____

8. To express regret (4)

_____

A	AV	CA	CON
COOK	DI	DO	DO
E	E	EN	GEN
GIZE	I	IE	MIN
NO	O	O	OPE
POL	SAURS	SION	SIS
TEL	UM	VEL	VI

Answers on page 333

Griddle

Find as many words with four or more connected letters as you can in two minutes. The letters must touch either vertically, horizontally, or diagonally. You cannot skip or jump across letters and you cannot use the same letter twice in one word. For example, to make the word *loyal*, you must have two Ls in the grid. Proper nouns are not allowed.

O	R	T	S
A	E	Y	O
L	S	B	L
C	S	U	E

_____   _____   _____

_____   _____   _____

_____   _____   _____

_____   _____   _____

_____   _____   _____

_____   _____   _____

_____   _____   _____

_____   _____   _____

_____   _____   _____

_____   _____   _____

_____   _____   _____

_____   _____   _____

_____   _____   _____

_____   _____   _____

_____   _____   _____

_____   _____   _____

_____   _____   _____

Answers on page 334

OPPOSITES
ATTRACT

Rearrange the letters of each word provided to reveal a pair of opposite words.

1. Aft/Hint   _____   _____

2. Rifts/Salt   _____   _____

3. Pats/Serpent   _____   _____

4. Peed/Hallows   _____   _____

5. Malls/Glare   _____   _____

Answers on page 334

Four Tricky Tongue Twisters!

Repeat each tongue twister three times quickly and out loud, without making a mistake.

A black bug's blood

A cricket critic

Mixed biscuits

Betty better butter bread

HIDDEN QUOTATION

Cross out all words on the next page as instructed below. Then rearrange the remaining words (those that were not crossed out) to reveal a quotation from Winston Churchill.

1. Cross out the names of all countries in Asia.

2. Cross out the last names of all actors from the TV show *Cheers*.

3. Cross out all names of Snow White's dwarfs (Disney version).

4. Cross out all misspelled words.

5. Cross out the names of all presidential cabinet departments.

6. Cross out all units of measurement.

long-term memory,
working memory,
attention to detail,
executive functioning

JAPAN	HELL	GRUMPY	ALLEY
BUISINESS	LONG	IRAN	BELEIVE
YOU'RE	MILE	STICHES	LABOR
DOPEY	ENERGY	CUP	GREATFUL
GOING	DOC	IF	INDIA
GOING	YARD	STATE	THROUGH
WENDT	KEEP	OMAN	DANSON

Quotation:

_____

_____

_____

Answers on page 334

HAPPY ENDINGS

working memory,
multitasking,
attention to detail

Can you come up with the missing letters that complete each set of words? Here's an example:

| CA____ | SWE____ | OBSE____ | CONSE____ |

The correct answer is **RVE** (**CARVE, SWERVE, OBSERVE, CONSERVE**).

1	PO___	GENE___	NUME___	VIGO___
2	LA____	ENO____	THRO___	HICCO___
3	VA____	OCC____	RES____	ASSA____
4	RE____	ASS____	FORE____	CAMPA___

Answers on page 334

Riddle Me This

Classic riddles like this one are easier to solve if you think outside the box.

....

How many three-cent stamps are in a dozen?

....

Answer on page 334

Making Connections

Given six words in the grid, can you find the three pairs that belong together and explain why each is a pair?

ZIP	DASH
ESCORT	NADA
COLON	PINTO

In the sample above, one pair is *Escort* and *Pinto*, which are both Ford car models. Another pair is *Zip* and *Nada*, which both mean *nothing*. And *Dash* and *Colon* are both punctuation marks.

HUD	3^2
SAT	IX
DOJ	WED

Pair_____   Theme _____

Pair_____   Theme _____

Pair_____   Theme _____

Answers on page 334

Join 'Em

Join together any two words from the columns on the left below, putting an L in the middle, to create one longer word. For example: *EMU* plus *ATE* with an *L* in the middle is *EMULATE*. While there might be alternates, only one way works for all the words. *Note: The shorter words can come from the same column or both columns.*

SHORT WORDS		LONGER WORDS
ACES	ASH	1 _____ L _____
BOX	EDGE	2 _____ L _____
EYE	ID	3 _____ L _____
IMP	KNOW	4 _____ L _____
ORE	SHOE	5 _____ L _____
SO	TOO	6 _____ L _____

Answers on page 335

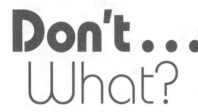

Don't...
What?

We found twenty-two well-known proverbs or sayings that begin with the word *Don't*. How many can you come up with in two minutes? (Get five and you're doing great!)

_____

_____

_____

_____

_____

_____

_____

_____

_____

_____

Answers on page 335

Dog Eat Dog

The answer to each clue is a phrase or saying that contains the word DOG.

1. In trouble, especially with one's spouse

_____

2. A heavy downpour

_____

3. Everyone has success or good luck at some point in their lives

_____

4. Don't interfere in something that isn't causing a problem

_____

5. Only they go out "in the noonday sun"

_____

Answers on page 335

Letter Play

The goal of this game is to come up with the Letter Play Word at the bottom of the page. To do that, you must 1) finish each word in the list with the correct letter, chosen from the options in parentheses. Then 2) place that letter in the blank space of the Letter Play Word that corresponds with its clue number.

1. __ANDLE (C, H)

2. P__AYER (L, R)

3. __ARS (E, J)

4. PUR__E (G, S)

5. EXPLO__E (D, R)

6. GLO__E (B, V)

7. P__RCH (A, E)

8. M__STER (A, I)

__ __ __ __ __ __ __ __
5 3 1 8 6 7 2 4

Answers on page 335

Word Rebus

Each picture rebus represents a word. Pay close attention to the plus and minus signs to know which sound to add or remove.

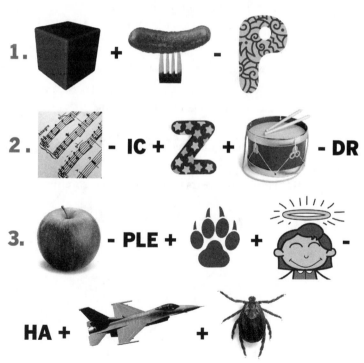

1. [cube] + [sausage] - [hanger]

2. [music] - IC + Z + [drum] - DR

3. [apple] - PLE + [paw] + [angel] -
HA + [jet] + [tick]

Answers on page 336

It's TIME!

long-term memory,
working memory

It's time to answer some questions about time.

1. How many days are in a fortnight?

2. How many years in a millennium?

3. How many months in a century?

4. How many years in four score and seven?

Answers on page 336

Change a Letter

long-term memory,
attention to detail,
multitasking,
executive functioning

Change the three given words into new words by replacing one letter—without rearranging any of the existing letters. For example: PLAY, SNAIL, WAIST can be changed to PRAY, SNARL, WRIST. You can change any one of the existing letters, but you must use the same replacement letter for all three words.

1. Arid, Incite, Lease

2. Butter, Driver, Filmed

3. Eat, Binge, Battle

4. Owes, Calmer, Scamp

Answers on page 336

It's All in the Name

In this two-part game, you must first answer the clues, then put the answers in the correct order to reveal the name of a famous person. Here's a sample question: *The sound of a growl + Men's neckwear + The forest.* The answers are: *Grr + Tie + Woods.* Rearrange those answers and you get *Tie + Grr + Woods.*

1. Door unlocker + Teams that row boats together + "Goodbye" or "Thanks" in London + A little shaving cut + A professional cook

2. 1960s baseball pitcher Mr. Drysdale + Body at the center of our solar system + Slang term for the toilet + Paul, who sat in the center of *Hollywood Squares* for years

3. "Open your mouth and say . . ." this + A place to sit in the park + To chop into tiny pieces + *Star Trek* character who is half Vulcan

Answers on page 336

DOUBLE TROUBLE

Given a list of words such as *knuckle*, *moth*, and *basket*, can you find the one word that follows each of them to make a compound word or a two-word phrase? For the example words above, the correct answer is *ball* (*knuckleball*, *mothball*, and *basketball*). *Note: The first letter of each answer is provided in a hint below . . . but try not to use it unless you're really stuck!*

In this special version of Double Trouble, all of the answers are ANIMALS.

1. Book, Silk, Tape

4. Talk, Cold, Wild

2. Eat, Jim, Scare

5. Spring, Rubber, Fried

3. Cry, Lone, Timber

(Hints: 1-W, 2-C, 3-W, 4-T, 5-C)

Answers on page 336

Identify This!

Can you match each somewhat uncommon word or phrase with its corresponding image?

SPORK

_____

BALACLAVA

_____

GEODUCK

_____

F-HOLE

_____

SCOTTISH FOLD

_____

KINKAJOU

_____

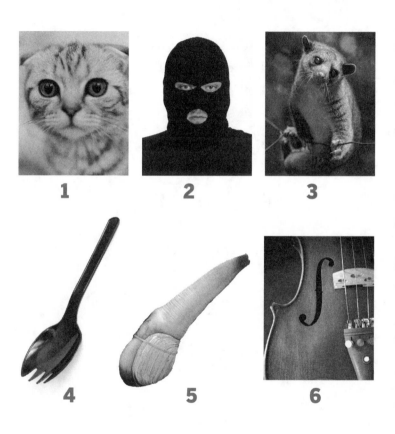

1

2

3

4

5

6

Answers on page 336

FLAG Words

long-term memory, attention to detail, executive functioning

Every word in this list is missing the letters F-L-A-G. Can you put those letters back (in any order) in the spaces below to reveal a common English word?

1. __ RU __ __ __

2. __ R __ __ I __ E

3. __ E __ P __ RO __

4. __ R __ TE __ U __

5. __ __ OOD __ __ TE

6. __ I __ E __ U __ RD

Answers on page 336

Riddle Me This

Classic riddles like this one are easier to solve if you think outside the box.

....

During what month do people sleep the least?

....

Answer on page 336

ODD MAN OUT

In each list of items, all but one have something in common. Can you find the item that doesn't belong AND explain why it is the Odd Man Out?

1. Cassiopeia, Orion, Scorpius, Cormorant

2. Shuttlecock, Shylock, Puck, Falstaff

3. Quiche, Vichyssoise, Borscht, Gazpacho

4. Lake Placid, Gettysburg, Baseball Hall of Fame, Coney Island

Answers on page 336

Saintly Things

Sometimes saints show up in unexpected places. Can you find the *saint* in these people, places, and things?

1. A brand of aspirin

2. Children's hospital founded by Danny Thomas

3. Hospital that's the setting for a 1980s TV series

4. Charles Lindbergh's airplane

5. Medicinal herb said to have antidepressant properties

6. Full and proper name for the Mormon church

Answers on page 337

Presidential Quotations

long-term memory,
working memory,
executive functioning

Can you match the quote with the US president who said it?

1. "Read my lips: no new taxes."

2. "You can fool all of the people some of the time, and some of the people all of the time, but you cannot fool all of the people all of the time."

3. "I think that this is the most extraordinary collection of talent, of human knowledge, that has ever been gathered together at the White House, with the possible exception of when Thomas Jefferson dined alone."

4. "This generation of Americans has a rendezvous with destiny."

a. Abraham Lincoln

b. Franklin D. Roosevelt

c. John F. Kennedy

d. George H.W. Bush

Answers on page 337

WORD TOWER

Build a tower of words that begins with the letters TA by increasing the number of letters in each consecutive word by one (example for the letters NO: NOT, NOON, NORTH, and so on). You cannot just add an S to a word already used, and no proper nouns are allowed. If you come up with words longer than eight letters, you're a Word Tower pro! *This game is a better brain booster if you put a one- or two-minute time limit on it.*

1. TA

2. TA __

3. TA __ __

4. TA __ __ __

5. TA __ __ __ __

6. TA __ __ __ __ __

7. TA __ __ __ __ __ __

8. TA __ __ __ __ __ __ __

Answers on page 337

OPPOSITES
ATTRACT

multitasking, executive functioning

Rearrange the letters of each word provided to reveal a pair of opposite words.

1. Desert/Tried _____ _____

2. Fats/Owls _____ _____

3. Vole/Heat _____ _____

4. Glean/Lived _____ _____

5. Baker/Rapier _____ _____

Answers on page 337

Four Tricky Tongue Twisters!

Repeat each tongue twister three times quickly and out loud, without making a mistake.

Santa's short suit shrunk

Fred's fresh flash message

Six clams crammed
in a clean cream can

Snap crackle pop

What's the Word?

Identify the missing letters that complete each row of words. For example, given the clues: ___ **NERS, AL___AC, HU___, ___SION,** the correct answer is *MAN (Manners, Almanac, Human, Mansion). Note: All missing letters will form a three-letter word.*

B _ _ _	SP _ _ _	T _ _ _ ET	TURM _ _ _
IS _ _ _	TIS _ _ _	_ _ _ DE	PUR _ _ _
_ _ _ K	S _ _ _ K	_ _ _ KET	FRAN _ _ _
DI _ _ _	_ _ _ ITY	AD _ _ _ CE	_ _ _ ILLA

Answers on page 337

EIGHTS & Fours

Can you make one eight-letter word and two four-letter words from the scrambled letters below?

1.

A E O B D R R W

_ _ _ _ _ _ _ _

_ _ _ _

_ _ _ _

2.

A A E B B L L S

_ _ _ _ _ _ _ _

_ _ _ _

_ _ _ _

Answers on page 337

Picture Connections

Find the three groups of three related pictures and explain why they are connected. For example, if three of the nine pictures were *Johnny Carson*, *Jay Leno*, and *Jimmy Fallon*, they would be connected as *Tonight Show hosts*.

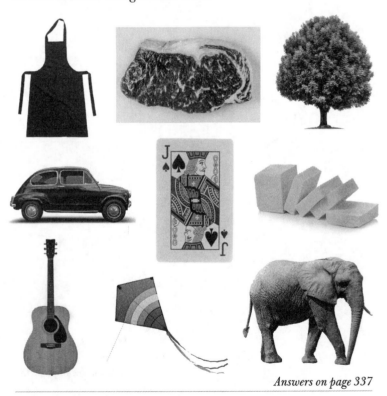

Answers on page 337

Give Me a Word That . . .

working memory, multitasking, attention to detail, processing speed

You can make this into an especially challenging brain exercise if you answer each question completely within one minute.

1. Give me four words that . . . contain the letter Q, but NOT in the first position.

_____

2. Give me three five-letter words that . . . have only one vowel.

_____

3. Give me four words or phrases that . . . mean *sick*.

_____

Answers on page 337

One-Minute Madness

How many single words that complete the compound word or two-word phrase _____ WATER can you name in one minute? (If you come up with more than ten, you're doing great!)

_____

_____

_____

_____

_____

_____

_____

_____

_____

_____

_____

Answers on page 338

JiNGLES & SLOGANS

Finish the jingle or advertising slogan, and then name the product (unless it's already named in the answer).

1. "Maybe she's born with it, _____."

_____

2. "It's the quicker _____."

_____

3. "Nobody doesn't like _____."

_____

4. "What would you do for _____?"

_____

5. "If you've got the time, we've _____."

_____

Answers on page 338

Pictures
& Parts

By combining one picture and one partial word, can you come up with the names of six foods? For example, a picture of a *flower* plus the partial word *cauli* makes *cauliflower*. *Note: The spelling may not always be exact, but the pronunciation will always be correct.*

COO	SAGE	EW
BO	BROW	ARTI

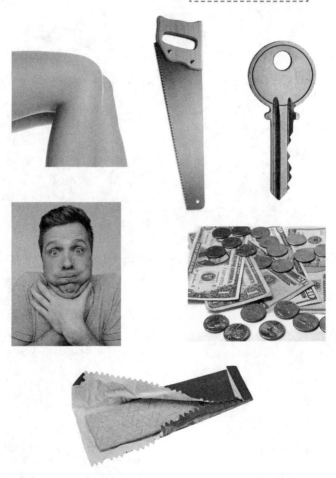

Answers on page 338

CHAPTER FIVE

Hang Tough!

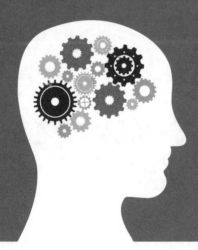

Is or Isn't?

long-term memory, working memory, executive functioning

In this game, you have to find the one item in each list that is—or isn't—what we say it is . . . or isn't.

1. Which one is . . . a car model?
   a. Cheetah   **b.** Antelope
   c. Rabbit   **d.** Tiger

2. Which isn't . . . a breakfast cereal?
   a. Cookie Crisp   **b.** Brownie Bits
   c. Crispix   **d.** Honey Smacks

3. Which city is . . . in Massachusetts?
   a. Providence   **b.** Provincetown
   c. Portland   **d.** Penobscot

4. Which line is . . . found in the Bible?
   a. To thine own self be true.
   b. To everything there is a season.
   c. Familiarity breeds contempt.
   d. Ask no questions and you'll be told no lies.

Answers on page 338

Wacky Wordy

The arrangement of the letters in the frame is a clue to the answer. For example, if the word *school* were placed high up in the frame, the answer would be *high school*. Or if the phrase *easy pieces* occurred five times in the frame, the answer would be *five easy pieces*.

Sympho . . .

Answer on page 338

TWO BY THREE

In this game, a three-letter word determines what your two answers can be. Let's take the word *WAD*, for example. If the first question is: *Name two authors for each letter*, the answers might be: **W**: *Thornton Wilder and H. G. Wells*, **A**: *Louisa May Alcott and Maya Angelou*, **D**: *Charles Dickens and Joan Didion*.

1. Come up with two one-syllable words that start with each letter (and have at least four letters).

2. Name two colors that start with each letter.

3. Name two countries that start with each letter.

	One-Syllable Words	Colors	Countries
H			
I			
T			

Answers on page 338

Common Bonds

long-term memory,
multitasking,
attention to detail

Find the common bond (or theme) among three very different pictures.

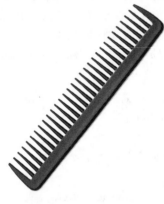

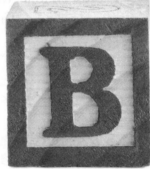

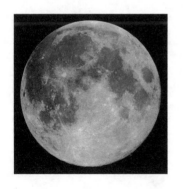

Answer on page 338

Endings & Beginnings

In this game, we provide the first half of one compound word or two-word phrase and the second half of another. Can you come up with the one word that completes both? *Note: The first letter of each answer is provided in a hint below . . . but try not to use it unless you're really stuck!*

1. Pony _____ Gate

2. Watch _____ Fight

3. Type _____ Lift

4. Space _____ Agent

5. Hang _____ Polish

SECRET

Word

How many four- or five-letter words can you find using the letters in the phrase below? The more words you find, the more likely you are to discover the secret word, which is generally a little harder to spot. (It's designated in the Solutions section.) To make this game a better brain exercise, try to find at least a dozen words in one minute.

IDAHO POTATO

_____	_____	_____	_____
_____	_____	_____	_____
_____	_____	_____	_____
_____	_____	_____	_____
_____	_____	_____	_____
_____	_____	_____	_____
_____	_____	_____	_____
_____	_____	_____	_____

Answers on page 339

Mathematically
Speaking

long-term memory,
working memory

Although the questions in this quiz have little or nothing to do with math, all of the answers do. For example, the answer to the clue *An Egyptian burial tomb* is *pyramid*—which, mathematically speaking, is a geometric shape.

1. In the 1950s and 1960s, this was the opposite of a "hip" person.

2. What a pilot does if there are too many airplanes trying to land.

3. A unit of ice.

4. A measure of the percentage of alcohol content in whiskey, gin, and other hard liquors.

5. This percussion instrument is very popular in grammar school bands.

Answers on page 339

HIDDEN QUOTATION

Cross out all words on the next page as instructed below. Then rearrange the remaining words (those that were not crossed out) to reveal a quotation from Abraham Lincoln.

1. Cross out all words that start with a silent letter.

2. Cross out all beverages.

3. Cross out all things that have wheels.

4. Cross out words that begin and end with the twelfth letter of the alphabet.

5. Cross out all Roman numerals.

6. Cross out all senses.

long-term memory,
working memory,
attention to detail,
executive functioning

C	LEVEL	ARE	KNIFE
ONE	LIBEL	TOUCH	WATER
PSALM	A	IX	WHATEVER
SODA	JUICE	YOU	BICYCLE
BUS	GOOD	BE	AISLE
WRITER	LEGAL	M	TASTE

Quotation:

_____

_____

_____

Answers on page 339

Stinky Pinky

Each Stinky Pinky answer contains two words that rhyme. Can you figure out what that answer is from an offbeat definition? For example, the answer to the clue *Mrs. Onassis's tan pants* is *Jackie's khakis*.

1. The entrance to a house in Oslo

2. A cantaloupe that was convicted of a crime

3. A tasty marine crustacean that is a member of the mafia

4. An inn for a small antelope

5. Plates for a flounder

Answers on page 339

Join 'Em

working memory, multitasking, attention to detail, executive functioning

Join together any two words from the columns on the left below, putting a T in the middle, to create one longer word. For example: *ASH* plus *RAY* with a *T* in the middle is *ASHTRAY*. *Note: The shorter words can come from the same column or both columns.*

SHORT WORDS		LONGER WORDS
BOOM	BRUSH	1 ____ T ____
BURN	CAP	2 ____ T ____
FOX	GEMS	3 ____ T ____
HEAR	ION	4 ____ T ____
ONE	OWN	5 ____ T ____
PAIN	ROT	6 ____ T ____

Answers on page 339

Run the Alphabet

From *Auto* to *Zero*, we're looking for a WORD THAT ENDS IN O for each letter of the alphabet. This game is a better brain booster if you put a two- or three-minute timer on it.

A_____   H_____   O_____   V_____

B_____   I_____   P_____   W_____

C_____   J_____   Q_____   X _(none)_

D_____   K_____   R_____   Y_____

E_____   L_____   S_____   Z_____

F_____   M_____   T_____

G_____   N_____   U_____

Answers on page 339

Geographical Nicknames

Can you identify each city by its nickname?

1. The Big Peach   _____

2. The Forbidden City   _____

3. Second City   _____

4. Witch City   _____

5. The Big Pineapple   _____

Answers on page 340

You Can't . . . What?

We found sixteen well-known proverbs or sayings that begin with the words *You can't* _____. How many can you come up with in two minutes? (Get five and you're doing great!)

_____

_____

_____

_____

_____

_____

_____

_____

_____

Answers on page 340

Sentence Sleuth

A true Sentence Sleuth can find the name of a DANCE (of any type) hidden somewhere in each of these sentences. The correct answer could be spread over more than one word, and all punctuation, capital letters, etc., should be ignored.

1. After the storm ended, I heard my mother shout, "Walt, zip up your parka and go shovel the driveway now!"

2. When a whale damaged his boat, Jim had to climb over the side and jump into the rubber raft.

3. Harry is a sports nut. He's always playing hockey, golf, tennis, basketball, etc.

Answers on page 340

NUMBER Words

multitasking, attention to detail, executive functioning

Just insert a numeral in the blank space to complete the word. For example, the correct answer to the clue *Lieu_____ant* is *Lieu 10 ant*.

1. Be _____

2. Sk _____

3. _____ th

4. _____ k

5. Ba _____

Answers on page 340

One-Minute Madness

How many OCCUPATIONS THAT BEGIN WITH THE LETTER "S" can you name in one minute? (If you come up with more than a dozen, you're doing great!)

Answers on page 340

CODE Words

long-term memory, attention to detail, executive functioning

Every word in this list is missing the letters C-O-D-E. Can you put those letters back (in any order) in the spaces below to reveal a common English word?

1. __ __ M __ __Y

2. S __ __ __ N __

3. __ __ N __ __ MN

4. __ H __ W __ __ R

5. __ __ U __ ATI __ N

6. ANN __ UN __ __ __

Answers on page 341

WORD TOWER

long-term memory,
processing speed,
executive functioning

Build a tower of words that begins with the letters HA by increasing the number of letters in each consecutive word by one (example for the letters NO: NOT, NOON, NORTH, and so on). You cannot just add an S to a word already used, and no proper nouns are allowed. If you come up with words longer than eight letters, you're a Word Tower pro! *This game is a better brain booster if you put a one- or two-minute time limit on it.*

1. HA

2. HA __

3. HA __ __

4. HA __ __ __

5. HA __ __ __ __

6. HA __ __ __ __ __

7. HA __ __ __ __ __ __

8. HA __ __ __ __ __ __ __

Answers on page 341

SAY WHAT?

Saul loves sayings and proverbs . . . but he can never remember them correctly. Can you fix his mistakes to reveal the correct saying? For example, Saul might say: "Humans who reside in clear, vitreous residences ought not to hurl small rocks." But the correct saying is: "People who live in glass houses should not throw stones."

1. "Refrain from severing your olfactory organ in order to defy your visage."

_____

2. "One-sixteenth of a pint's worth of avoidance is as valuable as sixteen ounces of complete healing."

_____

3. "The hardest gemstones are a young female's closest companion."

_____

4. "Place your currency in the same location as your oral cavity."

_____

5. "The most excellent item after carved brioche."

_____

Answers on page 341

Addables

long-term memory, multitasking, attention to detail

Each clue in *Addables* contains a word with a success scale in parentheses. The goal is to make as many new words as possible in two minutes by adding one letter and scrambling all the letters. With RUG, we found eight correct answers: **B**URG, **D**RUG, **F**RUG, GRU**B**, GUR**U**, RUG**S**, RU**N**G, U**R**GE.

The success scale for RUG is 4 out of 8, which means that if you get four correct answers, you are doing well. Get more, and you're an Addable Expert! The second number indicates the total number of common English words we found for that clue.

1. SIR   (9 out of 16)

2. NUT   (5 out of 11)

3. ACHE   (6 out of 12)

Answers on page 341

Griddle

Find as many words with four or more connected letters as you can in two minutes. The letters must touch either vertically, horizontally, or diagonally. You cannot skip or jump across letters and you cannot use the same letter twice in one word. For example, to make the word *loyal*, you must have two Ls in the grid. Proper nouns are not allowed.

D	L	T	A
O	R	I	M
W	Z	A	R
E	E	I	D

_____   _____   _____

_____   _____   _____

_____   _____   _____

_____   _____   _____

_____   _____   _____

_____   _____   _____

_____   _____   _____

_____   _____   _____

_____   _____   _____

_____   _____   _____

_____   _____   _____

_____   _____   _____

_____   _____   _____

_____   _____   _____

Answers on page 341

HAPPY ENDINGS

working memory, multitasking, attention to detail

Can you come up with the missing letters that complete each set of words? Here's an example:

| CA____ | SWE____ | OBSE____ | CONSE____ |

The correct answer is **RVE** (**CARVE, SWERVE, OBSERVE, CONSERVE**).

1	AP____	MA____	SIM____	STEE____
2	ST____	INF____	CONF____	UNIF____
3	P____	SW____	TW____	BEW____
4	BU____	WOO____	FINA____	CASUA____

Answers on page 341

Word Rebus

multitasking,
attention to detail,
executive functioning

Each picture rebus represents a word. Pay close attention to the plus and minus signs to know which sound to add or remove.

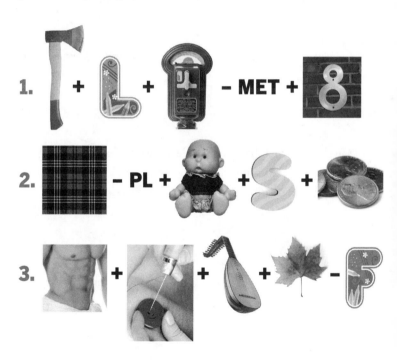

Answers on page 342

Give Me a Word That . . .

working memory,
multitasking,
attention to detail,
processing speed

You can make this into an especially challenging brain exercise if you answer each question completely within one minute.

1. Give me two words that . . . mean *hello* in any language other than English.

2. Give me five words that . . . have only one consonant.

3. Give me a word that . . . has at least two different meanings. For example: *Bat* (an animal and a piece of baseball equipment) or *Bark* (a tree covering and a dog sound).

Answers on page 342

ODD MAN OUT

long-term memory,
working memory,
executive functioning

In each list of items, all but one have something in common. Can you find the item that doesn't belong AND explain why it is the Odd Man Out?

1. Under, Either, Over, Around

2. Burr, Eisenhower, Humphrey, Mondale

3. Puerto Rico, Grand Cayman, Cyprus, Aruba

4. *Desk Set, Woman of the Year, Guess Who's Coming to Dinner, The Big Sleep*

Answers on page 342

EIGHTS & Fours

Can you make one eight-letter word and two four-letter words from the scrambled letters below?

1.
E A G G N S T R

— — — — — — — —

— — — —

— — — —

2.
A A E D D M R Y

— — — — — — — —

— — — —

— — — —

Answers on page 342

Letter Play

The goal of this game is to come up with the Letter Play Word at the bottom of the page. To do that, you must 1) finish each word in the list with the correct letter, chosen from the options in parentheses. Then 2) place that letter in the blank space of the Letter Play Word that corresponds with its clue number.

1. L__ST   (O, U)

2. S__Y   (A, L)

3. STA__LE   (B, P)

4. CAL__ER   (L, M)

5. DO__S   (E, G)

6. __IGHT   (L, R)

__ __ __ __ __ __
6   1   4   3   2   5

Answers on page 342

Four Tricky Tongue Twisters!

Repeat each tongue twister three times quickly and out loud, without making a mistake.

Black background,
brown background

Stupid superstition

Watch Rich risk all

Frank's friend flips fine flapjacks

Making Connections

Given six words in the grid, can you find the three pairs that belong together and explain why each is a pair?

ZIP	DASH
ESCORT	NADA
COLON	PINTO

In the sample above, one pair is *Escort* and *Pinto*, which are both Ford car models. Another pair is *Zip* and *Nada*, which both mean *nothing*. And *Dash* and *Colon* are both punctuation marks.

BS	PI
MU	MI
VI	JD

Pair_____   Theme _____

Pair_____   Theme _____

Pair_____   Theme _____

Answers on page 342

Syllability

The answers to the questions below are made up only of syllables found in the grid. Cross out the syllables as you use them. The number in parentheses indicates the number of syllables in the answer.

1. Relating to an educational institution or scholarly person (4)

_____

2. A man eater (literally) (3)

_____

3. A young person with a tendency to commit crimes, usually minor (3)

_____

4. Fruits and vegetables, collectively (2)

_____

5. Intensely deep, bright, or clear (2)

_____

6. An inoculation (3)

_____

7. Awful, terrible, dreadful (3)

_____

long-term memory,
multitasking,
attention to detail,
executive functioning

8. Items to be bought or sold, goods, wares (3)

_____

9. The field of medicine concerned with skin diseases (5)

_____

A	AC	BAL	BLE
CAN	CHAN	DE	DEM
DER	DISE	DUCE	GY
HOR	IC	ID	IN
JEC	LIN	MA	MER
NI	O	PRO	QUENT
RI	TION	TOL	VIV

Answers on page 342

Scrambled States

Unscramble the letters in these unusual phrases to reveal the name of a US state. You can make this a better brain workout if you can unscramble all the state names in two minutes!

1. A HEN WHIMPERS _____

2. AAA LAMB _____

3. RAN MADLY _____

4. I'M ACHING _____

5. HAIRCUT SALOON _____

Answers on page 343

OPPOSITES

ATTRACT

Rearrange the letters of each word provided to reveal a pair of opposite words.

1. Seat/Stew   _____ _____

2. Tacit/Recall   _____ _____

3. Binge/Den   _____ _____

4. Ulcer/Dink   _____ _____

5. Finder/Yemen   _____ _____

Answers on page 343

TWO BY THREE

working memory, multitasking, attention to detail, processing speed

In this game, a three-letter word determines what your two answers can be. Let's take the word *WAD*, for example. If the first question is: *Name two authors for each letter*, the answers might be: **W**: *Thornton Wilder and H. G. Wells*, **A**: *Louisa May Alcott and Maya Angelou*, **D**: *Charles Dickens and Joan Didion*.

1. Name two jobs/occupations that start with each letter.

2. Name two body parts that start with each letter.

3. Name two birds that start with each letter.

	Jobs	Body Parts	Birds
G			
E			
M			

Answers on page 343

Change a Letter

long-term memory,
attention to detail,
multitasking,
executive functioning

Change the three given words into new words by replacing one letter—without rearranging any of the existing letters. For example: PLAY, SNAIL, WAIST can be changed to P<u>R</u>AY, SNA<u>R</u>L, W<u>R</u>IST. You can change any one of the existing letters, but you must use the same replacement letter for all three words.

1. Valve, Empire, Revenge _____ _____ _____

2. Pout, Whittle, Quartz _____ _____ _____

3. Two, Why, Spar _____ _____ _____

4. Urine, Lame, Cured _____ _____ _____

Answers on page 343

Picture Titles

long-term memory,
multitasking,
attention to detail,
executive functioning

Can you figure out three movie titles by combining two images below? Each image will be used only once.

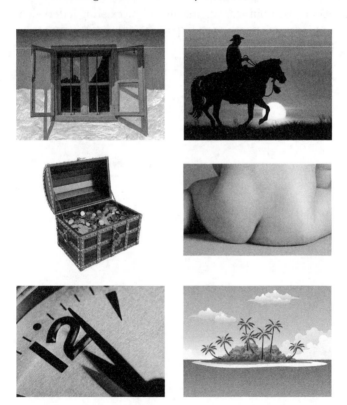

Answers on page 343

Order, Please!

long-term memory, working memory, multitasking, executive functioning

Given a list of three or four items, your job is to rearrange them in the order called for in the question.

1. According to *Forbes* magazine, these are among the top 50 highest-paying jobs in the United States. Put them in order, from highest-earning to lowest:

   ____ Nurse practitioner

   ____ Podiatrist

   ____ Pharmacist

2. Put these Monopoly properties in order by price, from lowest to highest:

   ____ Marvin Gardens

   ____ Tennessee Ave.

   ____ Indiana Ave.

Answers on page 343

KIND
Words

long-term memory, attention to detail, executive functioning

Every word in this list is missing the letters **K-I-N-D**. Can you put those letters back (in any order) in the spaces below to reveal a common English word?

1. __ __ __ __ EY

2. __ UC __ L __ __ G

3. WR __ __ __ LE __

4. QU __ C __ SA __ __

5. CA __ __ LEST __ C __

6. W __ __ __ BREA __ ER

Answers on page 343

Sentence Sleuth

A true Sentence Sleuth can find the name of a COUNTRY hidden somewhere in each of these sentences. The correct answer could be spread over more than one word, and all punctuation, capital letters, etc., should be ignored.

1. My brother Cliff ran Central City Cinema until it burned down.

2. "Using the hibachi," Lester said, "is the same as cooking on a barbecue grill."

3. Today I went to the kitchen store and bought a total of two pots, one pan, a Maytag dishwasher, and a Waring blender.

Answers on page 343

Riddle Me This

Classic riddles like this one are easier to solve if you think outside the box.

....

A cowboy rode to the nearest city on Friday. He stayed two nights and left on Friday. How could that be?

....

Answer on page 344

It's All in the Name

long-term memory, multitasking, executive functioning

In this two-part game, you must first answer the clues, then put the answers in the correct order to reveal the name of a famous person. Here's a sample question: *The sound of a growl* + *Men's neckwear* + *The forest*. The answers are: *Grr* + *Tie* + *Woods*. Rearrange those answers and you get *Tie* + *Grr* + *Woods*.

1. WWII diary keeper Miss Frank + The twelfth letter of the alphabet + Entrepreneur Mr. Zuckerberg + Ms. Ryan, costar of *Sleepless in Seattle*

2. Female horse + Fifth letter of the alphabet + A piece of evidence used to solve a crime + Uses oars + Large leg joint

3. President Reagan, for short + Mr. Brown, the "Godfather of Soul" + Where a research scientist usually works

Answers on page 344

Run the Alphabet

From *All in the Family* to *ZOOM*, we're looking for the TITLE OF A TV SHOW (past or present) for each letter of the alphabet. *Note: Disregard the initial* The, An, *or* A *in any titles.* The Rifleman, *for example, could be used for the letter R.* This game is a better brain booster if you put a two- or three-minute timer on it.

A_____ H_____ O_____ V_____

B_____ I_____ P_____ W_____

C_____ J_____ Q_____ X_____

D_____ K_____ R_____ Y_____

E_____ L_____ S_____ Z_____

F_____ M_____ T_____

G_____ N_____ U_____

Answers on page 344

Picture

Connections

Find the three groups of three related pictures and explain why they are connected. For example, if three of the nine pictures were *Johnny Carson*, *Jay Leno*, and *Jimmy Fallon*, they would be connected as *Tonight Show hosts*.

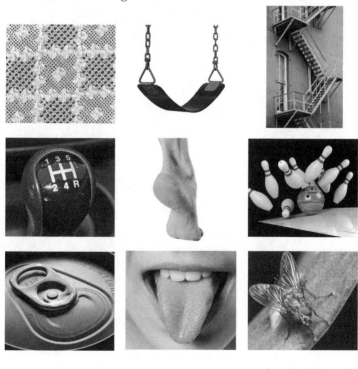

Answers on page 344

DOUBLE TROUBLE

Given a list of words such as *nip*, *burglar*, and *fish*, can you find the one word that precedes each of them to make a compound word or two-word phrase? For the example words above, the correct answer is *cat* (*catnip*, *cat burglar*, and *catfish*). *Note: The first letter of each answer is provided in a hint below . . . but try not to use it unless you're really stuck!*

1. Suit, Clerk, Firm

_____

2. Sake, Brand, Dropper

_____

3. Jury, Piano, Slam

_____

4. Elephant, Pages, Wash

_____

Need Directions?

long-term memory, working memory, multitasking

We provide the name of some of the most famous streets, intersections, and highways in the world, both real and fictional. Can you identify the city, country, region—or story—where each is located?

1. The Ginza   _____

2. Beale Street   _____

3. Lombard Street   _____

4. Gasoline Alley   _____

5. Khyber Pass   _____

6. Via Dolorosa   _____

Answers on page 344

What's the Word?

Identify the missing letters that complete each row of words. For example, given the clues: _ _ _ **NERS**, **AL** _ _ _ **AC**, **HU** _ _ _ , _ _ _ **SION**, the correct answer is *MAN* (*Manners, Almanac, Human, Mansion*). *Note: All missing letters will form a three-letter word.*

_ _ _ ORY	A _ _ _ IST	BREA _ _ _	CLO _ _ _ S
_ _ _ P	_ _ _ LL	A _ _ _ NG	PIG _ _ _ N
T _ _ _ P	F _ _ _ ED	_ _ _ BLE	CE _ _ _ IC
F _ _ _ S	A _ _ _ N	GOA _ _ _	RE _ _ _ F

Answers on page 344

Ted's Terrible Titles

Poor Ted. He is a connoisseur of culture, but he can never remember the titles of his favorite books, plays, songs, movies, etc. Can you fix Ted's mangled titles by correcting his mistakes?

1. From This Place Until Forever

_____

2. Gentle Be the Darkness

_____

3. Hubris and Bias

_____

4. The Summons of the Untamed

_____

5. Felony and Disciplinary Action

_____

6. Alabaster Long Pointed Tooth

_____

Answers on page 344

CHAPTER SIX

Finish Strong!

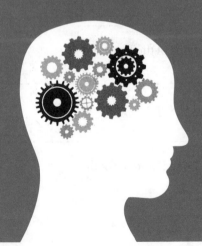

Give Me a Word That . . .

working memory, multitasking, attention to detail, processing speed

You can make this into an especially challenging brain exercise if you answer each question completely within one minute.

1. Give me five words that . . . begin with the letters KN.

2. Give me four words (or phrases) that . . . mean *drunk*.

3. Give me a word that . . . can be formed using all the letters in the word *ocean*.

Answers on page 345

HIDDEN QUOTATION

Cross out all words on the next page as instructed below. Then rearrange the remaining words (those that were not crossed out) to reveal a quotation from Albert Einstein.

1. Cross out all types of animals.

2. Cross out all men's names.

3. Cross out all last names of famous people whose first name is Joan.

4. Cross out all three-syllable words that start with a consonant.

5. Cross out all words that are names of car models.

6. Cross out all palindromes (words that read the same backward and forward).

long-term memory,
working memory,
attention to detail,
executive functioning

MADE	LEVEL	CAT	TRIED
NORMAN	RIVERS	NEW	WHO
TRIANGLE	NEVER	NOVA	LUNATIC
MISTAKE	ANDREW	A	RACCOON
MADAM	CAMRY	A	DART
PERSON	NEVER	BAEZ	ANYTHING
CRAWFORD	KAYAK	OWL	CANOPY

Quotation:

_____

_____

_____

Answers on page 345

FIND THE THEME

working memory, executive functioning

The list below contains anagrams of words that are all related to a theme. Unscramble the words, then determine the theme.

RATSZ

_____

EXFOWNS

_____

FLEETIMI

_____

VABOR

_____

PENS

_____

THEME:

_____

_____

Answers on page 345

One-Minute Madness

How many CARIBBEAN ISLANDS can you name in one minute?

_____

_____

_____

_____

_____

_____

_____

_____

_____

_____

Answers on page 345

Counting Syllables

long-term memory, multitasking, processing speed, executive functioning

Come up with the answers to these questions, syllable by syllable. Put a one-minute timer on each question and you'll get a better brain workout.

1. Name five musical instruments with three-syllable names.

2. Name three breakfast cereals with three-syllable names.

3. Name two world countries with one-syllable names.

4. Name the two months of the year with four-syllable names.

Answers on page 345

One-Minute Madness

long-term memory,
working memory,
processing speed

How many brands/types of COOKIES can you name in one minute?

_____

_____

_____

_____

_____

_____

_____

_____

_____

_____

Answers on page 346

People
Rebus

Each picture rebus below represents a famous person's name. Pay close attention to the plus and minus signs to know which sounds to add or remove.

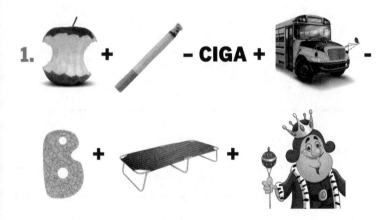

2. – NA + – EE +

3. + + C +

– + +

Answers on page 346

SAY WHAT?

Saul loves sayings and proverbs . . . but he can never remember them correctly. Can you fix his mistakes to reveal the correct saying? For example, Saul might say: "Humans who reside in clear, vitreous residences ought not to hurl small rocks." But the correct saying is: "People who live in glass houses should not throw stones."

1. "Do not take a nip from the palm and fingers that give you meals."

   _____

2. "The truth is the optimum political plan."

   _____

3. "Be optimistic for the superlative, get ready for the most unfavorable."

   _____

4. "No more quickly uttered than completed."

   _____

5. "You are able to guide a palomino to H_2O, but you are not able to compel him to imbibe."

   _____

Answers on page 346

WORD TOWER

Build a tower of words that begins with the letters WE by increasing the number of letters in each consecutive word by one (example for the letters NO: NOT, NOON, NORTH, and so on). You cannot just add an S to a word already used, and no proper nouns are allowed. If you come up with words longer than eight letters, you're a Word Tower pro! *This game is a better brain booster if you put a one- or two-minute time limit on it.*

1. WE

2. WE __

3. WE __ __

4. WE __ __ __

5. WE __ __ __ __

6. WE __ __ __ __ __

7. WE __ __ __ __ __ __

8. WE __ __ __ __ __ __ __

Answers on page 346

ODD MAN OUT

long-term memory,
working memory,
executive functioning

In each list of items, all but one have something in common. Can you find the item that doesn't belong AND explain why it is the Odd Man Out?

1. Garage, Guard, Hockey, Yard

2. Calabash, Wishbone, Corncob, Hookah

3. Delicious, Paris, Gala, Rome

4. Bolivia, Panama, Costa Rica, Guatemala

Answers on page 346

EIGHTS & Fours

working memory, multitasking, processing speed

Can you make one eight-letter word and two four-letter words from the scrambled letters below?

1. R T G H D A U E

_ _ _ _ _ _ _ _

_ _ _ _

_ _ _ _

2. T R U F A D I E

_ _ _ _ _ _ _ _

_ _ _ _

_ _ _ _

Answers on page 346

Pictures
& Parts

By combining one picture and one partial word, can you come up with six new words? For example, a picture of a *flower* plus the partial word *cauli* makes *cauliflower*. *Note: The spelling may not always be exact, but the pronunciation will always be correct.*

PION	ARIUM	INTRO
ASTRO	CON	ENNA

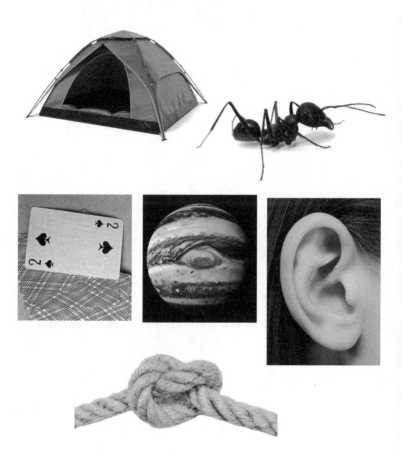

Answers on page 347

HIDDEN QUOTATION

Cross out all words on the next page as instructed below. Then rearrange the remaining words (those that were not crossed out) to reveal a quotation from W. C. Fields.

1. Cross out all furniture items.

2. Cross out all names of British prime ministers.

3. Cross out all items that are yellow.

4. Cross out all units of measurement.

5. Cross out all items that are typically made of glass.

long-term memory,
working memory,
attention to detail,
executive functioning

ARE	MAY	MIRROR	BUTTER
LEMON	IF	BLAIR	MILE
THEY	DESK	YARD	CHILDREN
METER	CORN	LIKE	LIGHTBULB
COOKED	I	INCH	THATCHER
BANANA	SOFA	WINDOW	PROPERLY

Quotation:

_____

_____

_____

Answers on page 347

Join 'Em

working memory, multitasking, attention to detail, executive functioning

Join together any two words from the columns on the left below, putting an S in the middle, to create one longer word. For example: *GOD* plus *END* with an *S* in the middle is *GODSEND*. *Note: The shorter words can come from the same column or both columns.*

SHORT WORDS		LONGER WORDS
BOMB	CORK	1 _____ S _____
CREW	DOME	2 _____ S _____
ELF	EYE	3 _____ S _____
GO	HELL	4 _____ S _____
HIM	ORE	5 _____ S _____
SIP	TIC	6 _____ S _____

Answers on page 347

COLORFILL

Put back the missing color in each phrase.

1. _____ parachute

2. _____ panther

3. Agent _____

4. _____ submarine

Answers on page 347

There's No . . . What?

We found 10 well-known proverbs or sayings that begin with the words *There's no* _____. How many can you come up with in two minutes? (Get four and you're doing great!)

_____

_____

_____

_____

_____

_____

_____

_____

_____

Answers on page 347

Do the Math!

working memory, multitasking, attention to detail

Do you remember the arithmetic you learned in school? It's time to exercise your math smarts by solving these problems.

Put the following sets of numbers in order from the smallest number to the largest:

$$\frac{5}{8} \qquad \frac{2}{6} \qquad \frac{1}{2}$$

$$\frac{13}{4} \qquad \frac{9}{2} \qquad \frac{16}{8}$$

$$.05 \qquad .1 \qquad .75 \qquad .15$$

Answers on page 347

QUOTATION STATION

Move the letters in each vertical column of the top grid to the column just below it in the bottom grid. Although the letters can only move down to the column below them, they will not necessarily be moved in the order in which they appear. If you move the letters to the correct positions, they will spell out a clever quotation from George Burns. *Note: A black square indicates the end of a word.*

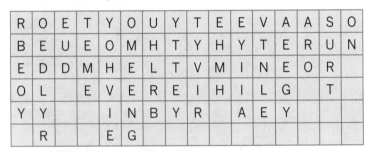

R	O	E	T	Y	O	U	Y	T	E	E	V	A	A	S	O
B	E	U	E	O	M	H	T	Y	H	Y	T	E	R	U	N
E	D	D	M	H	E	L	T	V	M	I	N	E	O	R	
O	L		E	V	E	R	E	I	H	I	L	G		T	
Y	Y			I	N	B	Y	R		A	E	Y			
	R			E	G										

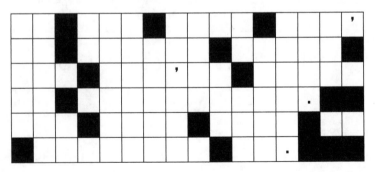

Answers on page 348

Who's Asking?

long-term memory,
working memory,
executive functioning

We provide the famous question. Can you identify who asked it?

1. "What did the president know and when did he know it?"

2. "Are you going to Scarborough Fair?"

3. "Is that all there is?"

4. "When it comes to establishing your worldview, what newspapers and magazines did you regularly read to stay informed?"

5. "Have you no sense of decency, sir? At long last, have you left no sense of decency?"

Answers on page 348

Change a Letter

long-term memory, attention to detail, multitasking, executive functioning

Change the three given words into new words by replacing one letter—without rearranging any of the existing letters. For example: PLAY, SNAIL, WAIST can be changed to P**R**AY, SNA**R**L, W**R**IST. You can change any one of the existing letters, but you must use the same replacement letter for all three words.

1. Wry, Sage, Brood _____ _____ _____

2. Fir, Coal, Edit _____ _____ _____

3. Wasted, Fabled, Grate _____ _____ _____

4. Accent, Commute, Suite _____ _____ _____

Answers on page 348

Riddle Me This

Classic riddles like this one are easier to solve if you think outside the box.

....

David's father has three sons named Tom, Dick, and _____?

....

Answer on page 348

DOUBLE TROUBLE

Given a list of words such as *nip*, *burglar*, and *fish*, can you find the one word that precedes each of them to make a compound word or two-word phrase? For the example words above, the correct answer is *cat* (*catnip*, *cat burglar*, and *catfish*). *Note: The first letter of each answer is provided in a hint below . . . but try not to use it unless you're really stuck!*

1. Collector, Bracket, Deduction

_____

2. Block, Map, Rage

_____

3. Belt, Order, Bags

_____

4. Muffin, Language, Teacher

_____

(Hints: 1-T, 2-R, 3-M, 4-E)

Answers on page 348

Sentence Sleuth

long-term memory,
multitasking,
attention to detail,
executive functioning

A true Sentence Sleuth can find the name of a FRUIT hidden somewhere in each of these sentences. The correct answer could be spread over more than one word, and all punctuation, capital letters, etc., should be ignored.

1. "Learn to play the tuba," Nana told Jason, "and you'll surely get a seat in the orchestra."

2. Joy told her worried Grandpa, "Pay a little each month, Pops, and they won't send a bill collector to your house."

3. After she realized that her students never heard of the Gestapo, Meg ran a teach-in about the Holocaust.

Answers on page 348

Word Rebus

Each picture rebus represents a word. Pay close attention to the plus and minus signs to know which sound to add or remove.

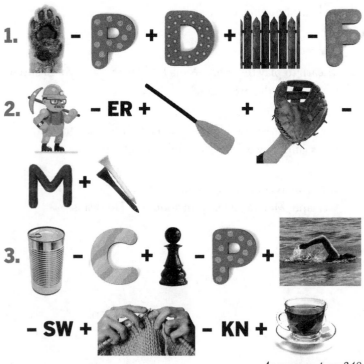

Answers on page 348

Whose
Biography?

Can you identify the famous subjects from the titles of their biographies, autobiographies, or memoirs? We've provided the years of their lives as a hint.

1. *A Moveable Feast* (1899–1961)

2. *I Know Why the Caged Bird Sings* (1928–2014)

3. *Kitchen Confidential* (1956–2018)

4. *The Long Walk to Freedom* (1918–2013)

5. *The Motorcycle Diaries: Notes on a Latin American Journey* (1928–1967)

Answers on page 348

Endings & Beginnings

working memory, multitasking

In this game, we provide the first half of one compound word or two-word phrase and the second half of another. Can you come up with the one word that completes both? *Note: The first letter of each answer is provided in a hint below . . . but try not to use it unless you're really stuck!*

1. Wall _____ Clip

2. Junk _____ Stamps

3. Holy _____ Town

4. Gold _____ Field

5. Track _____ Player

(*Hints: 1-P, 2-F, 3-G, 4-M, 5-R*)

Answers on page 349

SAY WHAT?

Saul loves sayings and proverbs . . . but he can never remember them correctly. Can you fix his mistakes to reveal the correct saying? For example, Saul might say: "Humans who reside in clear, vitreous residences ought not to hurl small rocks." But the correct saying is: "People who live in glass houses should not throw stones."

1. "I will traverse that raised road over water at the moment I arrive at it."

_____

2. "You are not able to hoodwink every person in every instance."

_____

3. "View you at a future time, large swamp-dwelling reptile."

_____

4. "The minutes take wing while you are participating in amusement."

_____

5. "If you can't be victorious over the others, unite with the others."

_____

Answers on page 349

Letter
Play

long-term memory,
multitasking,
attention to detail

The goal of this game is to come up with the Letter Play Word at the bottom of the page. To do that, you must 1) finish each word in the list with the correct letter, chosen from the options in parentheses. Then 2) place that letter in the blank space of the Letter Play Word that corresponds with its clue number.

1. P__LE   (I, O)

2. PA__PER   (M, U)

3. QUI__   (T, Z)

4. PA__TED   (R, S)

5. THE__E   (R, S)

__ __ __ __ __
5 3 1 4 2

Answers on page 349

Filled
with Emotion

The clues in this game are all phrases that contain an "emotional" word that is missing. For example: _____ Baby (*Melancholy* Baby) or Fighting _____ (Fighting *mad*). Can you put back the missing emotions?

1. Green with _____

2. Buyer's _____

3. _____ Club

4. Taken by _____

5. More's the _____

Answers on page 349

Fill In the Letters

long-term memory, attention to detail, processing speed, executive functioning

Fill in the blank spaces with letters to make common English words. (No proper nouns are allowed). For example, the clue __ **a t** yields twelve answers: *Bat, Cat, Eat, Fat, Hat, Mat, Oat, Pat, Rat, Sat, Tat, Vat. Note: The number in parentheses indicates how many common English words we found.* For a better cognitive workout, put a one-minute timer on each puzzle below.

1. D _ _ D   (5)

2. _ AN _ Y   (19)

Answers on page 349

What's the Animal?

All the answers in this game are two-word idioms or phrases that contain the name of an animal. We provide the first word. Can you come up with the animal?

1. Count _____

2. Cold _____

3. Play _____

4. Eat _____

5. Loan _____

6. Dark _____

Answers on page 349

It's All
in the Name

In this two-part game, you must first answer the clues, then put the answers in the correct order to reveal the name of a famous person. Here's a sample question: *The sound of a growl + Men's neckwear + The forest*. The answers are: *Grr + Tie + Woods*. Rearrange those answers and you get *Tie + Grr + Woods*.

1. To brown the skin by exposure to the sun + A web search engine/web services provider whose name includes an exclamation mark + Former Ugandan dictator Idi _____ + Tennis court divider + A place to sit at the park

2. Ice cream holder + The plural form of *is* + Dark viscous liquid derived from petroleum + Abbreviation for the day before Friday + Conjunction

3. Fifth letter of the alphabet + That thing + Tresses + Male adult + Fixture for bathing

Answers on page 349

One-Minute Madness

How many COUNTRIES WITH TWO-WORD NAMES can you name in one minute? (There are twenty-six of them, but you're doing exceptionally well if you get ten!)

_____

_____

_____

_____

_____

_____

_____

_____

_____

_____

_____

Answers on page 349

Sylla**bility**

The answers to the questions below are made up only of syllables found in the grid. Cross out the syllables as you use them. The number in parentheses indicates the number of syllables in the answer.

1. This killed the cat (5)

   _____

2. Flapjack (2)

   _____

3. Mr. Redenbacher's specialty (2)

   _____

4. Orange juice and vodka (3)

   _____

5. B_1 or B_{12} (3)

   _____

6. Multiplication, for example (4)

   _____

7. Mr. Webster's specialty (4)

   _____

8. Anderson Cooper or Shepard Smith (3)

long-term memory,
multitasking,
attention to detail,
executive functioning

_____

9. To remove a temporary fabric covering from a new monument or work of art as part of a public ceremony (2)

_____

A	AR	CAKE	CAST
CORN	CU	DIC	DRI
ER	I	ME	MIN
NEWS	OS	PAN	POP
RI	RITH	SCREW	TA
TIC	TION	TY	UN
VEIL	VER	VI	Y

Answers on page 350

EIGHTS & Fours

working memory,
multitasking,
processing speed

Can you make one eight-letter word and two four-letter words from the scrambled letters below?

1. AAECDLNR

_ _ _ _ _ _ _ _

_ _ _ _

_ _ _ _

2. AEUCFRRT

_ _ _ _ _ _ _ _

_ _ _ _

_ _ _ _

Answers on page 350

SECRET

Word

How many four- or five-letter words can you find using the letters in the word below? The more words you find, the more likely you are to discover the secret word, which is generally a little harder to spot. (It's designated in the Solutions section.) To make this game a better brain exercise, try to find at least a dozen words in one minute.

SPAGHETTI

Answers on page 350

Griddle

Find as many words with four or more connected letters as you can in two minutes. The letters must touch either vertically, horizontally, or diagonally. You cannot skip or jump across letters and you cannot use the same letter twice in one word. For example, to make the word *loyal*, you must have two Ls in the grid. Proper nouns are not allowed.

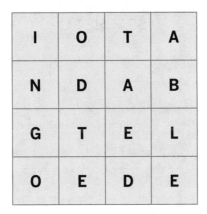

I	O	T	A
N	D	A	B
G	T	E	L
O	E	D	E

_____   _____   _____

_____   _____   _____

_____   _____   _____

_____   _____   _____

_____   _____   _____

_____   _____   _____

_____   _____   _____

_____   _____   _____

_____   _____   _____

_____   _____   _____

_____   _____   _____

_____   _____   _____

_____   _____   _____

_____   _____   _____

_____   _____   _____

_____   _____   _____

Answers on page 350

Four Tricky Tongue Twisters!

Repeat each tongue twister three times quickly and out loud, without making a mistake.

Fight French flu fast

_____

She wished for a Swiss wristwatch

_____

Will Fran flee from fog?

_____

Rolling red wagon

_____

WORD TOWER

Build a tower of words that begins with the letters DO by increasing the number of letters in each consecutive word by one (example for the letters NO: NOT, NOON, NORTH, and so on). You cannot just add an S to a word already used, and no proper nouns are allowed. If you come up with words longer than eight letters, you're a Word Tower pro! *This game is a better brain booster if you put a one- or two-minute time limit on it.*

1. DO

2. DO __

3. DO __ __

4. DO __ __ __

5. DO __ __ __ __

6. DO __ __ __ __ __

7. DO __ __ __ __ __ __

8. DO __ __ __ __ __ __ __

Answers on page 351

ODD MAN OUT

long-term memory, working memory, executive functioning

In each list of items, all but one have something in common. Can you find the item that doesn't belong AND explain why it is the Odd Man Out?

1. Oscar, Felix, Tony, Emmy

2. Bing, Reddit, Trident, Monster

3. Toronto, Michigan, Ontario, Erie

4. Shrimp, Chickens, Blessings, Calories

Answers on page 351

SAY WHAT?

Saul loves sayings and proverbs . . . but he can never remember them correctly. Can you fix his mistakes to reveal the correct saying? For example, Saul might say: "Humans who reside in clear, vitreous residences ought not to hurl small rocks." But the correct saying is: "People who live in glass houses should not throw stones."

1. "No male human is an area of land surrounded by water."

   _____

2. "The sooner-than-expected flying animal receives the fish bait."

   _____

3. "What you do articulates with more volume than vocabulary units."

   _____

4. "Not hard arrival, not hard departure."

   _____

5. "It is superior to be behind time than at no time."

   _____

Answers on page 351

Counting Syllables

Come up with the answers to these questions, syllable by syllable. Put a one-minute timer on each question and you'll get a better brain workout.

1. Name the three months of the year with two-syllable names.

2. Name three South American countries with four-syllable names.

3. Name four vegetables with one-syllable names.

4. Name four of the nine US presidents whose last names have one syllable.

Answers on page 351

Riddle Me This

Classic riddles like this one are easier to solve if you think outside the box.

····················

When can six large people fit under one small umbrella and not get wet?

····················

Answer on page 351

HAPPY ENDINGS

Can you come up with the missing letters that complete each set of words? Here's an example:

| CA___ | SWE____ | OBSE___ | CONSE___ |

The correct answer is **RVE** (**CARVE, SWERVE, OBSERVE, CONSERVE**).

1	AN____	BAD____	FIN____	SWIN___
2	C_____	SM_____	STR____	PROV___
3	GAL____	WAL____	DEVE____	SCAL____
4	PO____	REF____	COMPO___	PROFO__

Answers on page 351

TWO BY THREE

In this game, a three-letter word determines what your two answers can be. Let's take the word *WAD*, for example. If the first question is: *Name two authors for each letter,* the answers might be: **W**: *Thornton Wilder and H. G. Wells,* **A**: *Louisa May Alcott and Maya Angelou,* **D**: *Charles Dickens and Joan Didion.*

1. Name two vegetables that start with each letter.

2. Provide two boy's names that start with each letter.

3. Name two makes or models of automobiles that start with each letter.

	Vegetables	Boys' Names	Autos
L			
O			
P			

Answers on page 351

NUMBER

Words

Just insert a numeral in the blank space to complete the word.
For example, the correct answer to the clue *Lieu____ant* is
Lieu 10 ant.

1. Car _____ n

2. S _____ ch

3. Qui _____

4. _____ est

5. Or _____ or

Answers on page 352

Fill In the Letters

Fill in the blank spaces with letters to make common English words. (No proper nouns allowed.) For example, the clue __ **a t** yields twelve answers: *Bat, Cat, Eat, Fat, Hat, Mat, Oat, Pat, Rat, Sat, Tat, Vat. Note: The number in parentheses indicates how many common English words we found.* For a better cognitive workout, put a one-minute timer on each puzzle below.

1. MI __ __   (22)

2. __ __ GHT   (10)

Answers on page 352

Do the Math!

Probability is the mathematical likelihood that a particular event will occur. For example, the probability of tossing a coin and having it land on heads is 1 in 2, or 50 percent. See if you can calculate these probabilities.

1. What is the probability of rolling one standard die and getting the number 3?

2. What is the probability that you will pull a red card from a standard deck of 52 cards?

3. What is the probability that you will pull an ace from a standard deck of cards?

4. Which is more likely: tossing a coin and getting heads, or pulling a red card from a deck of cards?

Answers on page 352

Wacky Wordy

The arrangement of the letters in the frame is a clue to the answer. For example, if the word *school* were placed high up in the frame, the answer would be *high school*. Or if the phrase *easy pieces* occurred five times in the frame, the answer would be *five easy pieces*.

STEP
PETS
PETS

Answer on page 352

Sentence Sleuth

long-term memory,
multitasking,
attention to detail,
executive functioning

A true Sentence Sleuth can find the name of a BIRD hidden somewhere in each of these sentences. The correct answer could be spread over more than one word, and all punctuation, capital letters, etc., should be ignored.

1. "Mom," asked Heidi Finkle on the day before Thanksgiving, "can a rye or pumpernickel bread be used in stuffing?"

2. "Animal organs, such as heart, lungs, liver, or brains, are called offal," Connie said, "but I call them awful."

3. After the zebra ventured into the lion enclosure, the zoo staff scrambled to get him out.

Answers on page 352

DOUBLE TROUBLE

Given a list of words such as *nip*, *burglar*, and *fish*, can you find the one word that precedes each of them to make a compound word or two-word phrase? For the example words above, the correct answer is *cat* (*catnip*, *cat burglar*, and *catfish*). *Note: The first letter of each answer is provided in a hint below . . . but try not to use it unless you're really stuck!*

1. Alley, Date, Fold

3. Pilot, Drive, Tube

2. Story, Bread, Cut

4. Code, Service, Agent

(Hints: 1-B, 2-S, 3-T, 4-S)

Answers on page 352

Run the Alphabet

From *Auto racing* to *Zui quan (Drunken boxing)*, we're looking for the name of a SPORT OR OUTDOOR GAME for each letter of the alphabet. This game is a better brain-booster if you put a two- or three-minute timer on it.

A_____   H_____   **O** (obscure)   V_____

B_____   I_____   P_____   W_____

C_____   J_____   Q_____   **X** (obscure)

D_____   K_____   R_____   Y_____

E_____   L_____   S_____   **Z** (obscure)

F_____   M_____   T_____

G_____   N_____   U_____

Answers on page 352

What's the Word?

Identify the missing letters that complete each row of words. For example, given the clues: _ _ _ **NERS**, **AL**_ _ _ **AC**, **HU**_ _ _, _ _ _ **SION**, the correct answer is *MAN* (*Manners, Almanac, Human, Mansion*). *Note: All missing letters will form a three-letter word.*

CO _ _ _	_ _ _ IN	_ _ _ VEST	_ _ _ CELET
B _ _ _	WH _ _ _	BR _ _ _ H	CR _ _ _ URE
W _ _ _ D	DES _ _ _	ADM _ _ _	D _ _ _ CTOR
BUD _ _ _	NUG _ _ _	TAR _ _ _	VE _ _ _ ABLE

Answers on page 352

Riddle Me This

Classic riddles like this one are easier to solve if you think outside the box.

• • • • • • • • • • • • • • • • • • • •

One Sunday morning, a wealthy man was found dead in his mansion. When the police arrived, they started the investigation by interrogating the dead man's wife and the household staff. His wife said she was asleep. The cook said he was making breakfast. The gardener said he was picking vegetables. The maid said she was getting the morning mail. And the butler said he was cleaning the closet. When they were done, the police arrested the murderer. Whom did they arrest?

• • • • • • • • • • • • • • • • • • • •

Answer on page 352

One-Minute Madness

long-term memory,
working memory,
processing speed

How many of the TEN LARGEST US STATES (in area) can you come up with in one minute?

_____

_____

_____

_____

_____

_____

_____

_____

_____

_____

Answers on page 353

HIDDEN QUOTATION

Cross out all words on the next page that answer the questions below. Then rearrange the remaining words (those that were not crossed out) to reveal a quotation from famed football coach Vince Lombardi.

1. Cross out all words of three letters or more that rhyme with BOO.

2. Cross out all automobile makes or models.

3. Cross out all medical acronyms.

4. Cross out all brands of coffee.

5. Cross out all names of Native American tribes.

long-term memory,
working memory,
attention to detail,
executive functioning

THE	JUST	BMW	WE
OF	THROUGH	UTI	QUEUE
CLUE	LEXUS	NESCAFE	LOSE
OUT	WE	KIA	HOPI
FLU	KEURIG	APACHE	LOTUS
TIME	FOLGERS	DIDN'T	BP
GAME	CREE	RAN	GNU

Quotation:

_____

_____

_____

Answers on page 353

Give Me a Word That . . .

working memory, multitasking, attention to detail, processing speed

You can make this into an especially challenging brain exercise if you answer each question completely within one minute.

1. Give me a four-letter word that . . . has no anagrams (i.e., no other four-letter words can be made from the same letters). For example: *that* or *hoax*

2. Give me two words with five or more letters that . . . start with *cat*.

3. Give me two words with five or more letters that . . . end with *and*.

Answers on page 353

Picture Connections

Find the three groups of three related pictures and explain why they are connected. For example, if three of the nine pictures were *Johnny Carson*, *Jay Leno*, and *Jimmy Fallon*, they would be connected as *Tonight Show hosts*.

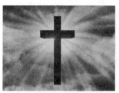
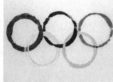
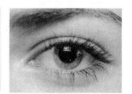

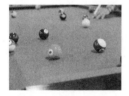
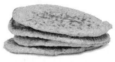
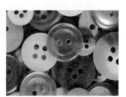

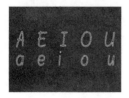
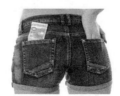
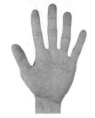

Answers on page 353

Solutions

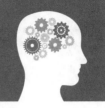

CHAPTER ONE

page 1: Is or Isn't?
1. (b) Leonardo DiCaprio
2. (c) Moolash
3. (d) Maple Tree Wilson
4. (b) Baghdad

page 2: What a Pair!
1. Wit and *wisdom*
2. Bits and *pieces*
3. *Hue* and cry
4. *Lock* and key
5. Part and *parcel*
6. Rules and *regulations*

page 3: Stinky Pinky
1. Crab lab
2. French stench
3. Phony pony
4. Sad dad
5. Funny money

page 4: Word Rebus
1. Poultry (Polo – O + Tree)
2. Diversity (Diver + City)
3. Cinderblock (Sink – K + Derby – Y + Lock)

page 5: What's the Word?
Lid   Valid, Collide, Solid, Holiday

Rob   Throb, Probate, Robot, Acrobat

Bed   Bedroom, Bombed, Climbed, Stabbed

Pan   Panther, Pantry, Pancreas, Occupant

page 6: Run the Alphabet: X Words

Appendix	Next
Box	Orthodox
Complex	Pixie
Dyslexic	Quixotic
Exit	Relax
Flexible	Saxophone
Galaxy	Tuxedo
Hoax	Unisex
Index	Vixen
Jinx	Wax
Kickboxer	Xylophone
Luxury	Y
Maximize	Z

page 7: Acronym Alphabet

1. Doctor of Veterinary Medicine
2. Earned run average/Equal Rights Amendment
3. First Lady of the United States
4. Point of view
5. Vehicle identification number
6. Oxford English Dictionary

page 8: Hidden Quotation

1. Area, Ironing, Aroma
2. Drum, Guitar, Flute, Cello
3. Lion, Yak, Frog
4. Crimson, Gray, Ecru
5. London, Seoul, Boston

Quotation: Don't regret the past; just learn from it.

page 10: Homonyms

1. Wail/Whale
2. Prey/Pray
3. Pour/Pore
4. Nose/Knows
5. Prophet/Profit

page 11: Riddle Me This

In the dictionary

page 12: What's the Animal?

1. Cash cow
2. Eager beaver
3. Grease monkey
4. Silly goose
5. Spring chicken
6. Dirty dog (Rat is also correct.)

page 13: Counting Syllables

(In some cases, other correct answers are possible.)

1. Eisenhower
2. Date, Fig, Grape, Lime, Peach, Pear, Plum
3. Alder, Apple, Aspen, Boxwood, Cedar, Cherry, Chestnut, Cypress, Dogwood, Maple, Olive, Pecan, Poplar, Redwood, Rosewood, Walnut, Willow
4. Bahrain, Belgium, Brazil, Chile, China, Congo, Cuba, Cyprus, Denmark, Egypt, Fiji, Finland, Georgia, Ghana, Haiti, Iceland, Iran, Iraq, Japan, Jordan, Kenya, Kuwait, Nepal, Norway, Oman, Peru, Poland, Qatar, Russia, Sweden, Taiwan, Thailand, Turkey, Ukraine, Yemen

page 14: Double Trouble

1. Water
2. Number
3. Girl
4. Head

page 15: Making Connections

Clues: Bobby, Knee
Theme: Socks

Clues: Gingrich, Blitzer
Theme: People whose first names are also animals (Newt Gingrich, Wolf Blitzer)

Clues: Junk, Fast
Theme: _____ food

page 16: One-Minute Madness: Dances

(Other correct answers are possible.)
Ballet, Ballroom, Barn dance, Belly dance, Bossa Nova, Break dance, Bunny Hop, Can Can, Cha Cha, Charleston, Clog, Conga, Contra dance, Country dance, Disco, Flamenco, Folk, Foxtrot, Frug, Hip-Hop, Hokey Pokey, Hora, Hully Gully, Hustle, Irish Jig, Jazz, Jitterbug, Jive, Limbo, Lindy Hop, Line dance, Macarena, Mambo, Merengue, Modern dance, Polka, Quickstep, Rain dance, Rumba, Salsa, Samba, Shimmy, Square dance, Swing, Tango, Tap, Twist, Vogue, Waltz

page 17: Change a Letter

(Other correct answers are possible.)
1. H: Flash, Why, Hour
2. E: Empire, Emit, Divine
3. U: Gum, Flu, Union
4. E: Brine, Then, Mange

page 18: Wacky Wordy

Cornerstone

page 19: Word Tower

(Other correct answers are possible.)
1. No
2. Now
3. Note
4. North
5. Noodle

6. Nothing
7. Nonsense
8. Novocaine

page 20: Jingles & Slogans

1. "... mouth, not in your hands."
   M&M's
2. "... light on for you."
   Motel 6
3. "... fit to print."
   the *New York Times*
4. "... positively has to be there overnight."
   FedEx
5. "... on earth."
   Disneyland

page 21: Fill In the Letters

(Other correct answers are possible.)
1. Brat, Brut, Drat, Frat, Fret, Grit, Trot, Writ
2. Daily, Dairy, Daisy, Deify, Deity, Doily

page 22: Common Bonds

Theme: Car models (Dart, Rabbit, Lincoln)

page 24: FINE Words

1. Knife
2. Benefit
3. Confide
4. Fifteen
5. Identify
6. Offensive

page 25: Order, Please!

1. Eiffel Tower (1,063'); Golden Gate Bridge (746'); Statue of Liberty (305')
2. Telescope (1608); Elevator (1853); Telephone (1876)

page 26: Say What?

1. Love makes the world go 'round.
2. Beggars can't be choosers.
3. If you can't be good, be careful.
4. Laughter is the best medicine.
5. There's no use beating a dead horse.

page 27: Animal Watching

A. Badger
B. Hyena
C. Anteater
D. Sloth

page 28: Riddle Me This

An egg

page 29: Down to the Wire

(Other correct answers are possible.)

1. *Dance* to the music
2. *Ear* to the ground
3. *Fly me* to the moon
4. *Race* to the top
5. *Shoulder* to the wheel

page 30: Eights & Fours

(Other correct answers are possible.)

1. Divorced   Cord/Dive
2. Floating   Gift/Loan

page 31: Pictures & People

Peter Graves
Emily Post
Joey Bishop
Al Capp
Larry Bird
Joan Rivers

page 32: Griddle

(Other correct answers are possible.)

4 Letters: Auto, Dean, Deed, Deem, Demo, Duet, Into, Meet, Mend, Mete, Mint, Moan, Moat, Mote, Need, Neon, None, Note, Omen, Teed, Teem, Teen, Tend, Toed, Tome, Tone

5 Letters: Anted, Atone, Demon, Eaten, Emote, Ended, Etude, Meted, Moted, Noted, Toned

6 Letters: Atoned, Demote, Denote, Emoted, Intend, Mended, Minted, Moated, Tended

7 Letters: Demoted, Denoted

8 Letters: Nominate, Intended

9 Letters: Nominated

10 Letters: Denominate

11 Letters: Denominated

page 34: Endings & Beginnings

1. Fool
2. Down
3. Cheese
4. Cross
5. Stick

page 35: Opposites Attract

1. Far/Near
2. Right/Left
3. North/South
4. Inside/Outside
5. Master/Servant

page 36: Hidden Quotation

1. Schwinn, Columbia, Huffy
2. Platinum, Gold, Silver
3. Carp, Perch, Guppy
4. Anonymous, Universal, Electrify
5. Lip, Toe, Knuckle
6. Globe, Post, Herald, Times, Tribune

Quotation: Silence is the best reply to a fool.

page 38: It's All in the Name

1. Car + E + Kim + Dash + In
   Kim Kardashian
2. Lane + E + Mick + Spill
   Mickey Spillane
3. Cah + Blow + Pick + Sew + Pa
   Pablo Picasso

page 39: Odd Man Out

1. Indianapolis is the odd man out. It is the capital of Indiana. All the rest are capitals of states with names that start with "New": New York, New Jersey, New Mexico.
2. Hello is the odd man out. All the other terms represent endings: Period (the end of a sentence), Z (the end of the alphabet), New Year's Eve (the end of the year), Amen (the end of a prayer).
3. CIA is the odd man out. It is a US federal agency. The other acronyms are all related to computers.
4. Telephone is the odd man out. All the others are types of cups.

page 40: What's the Word?

Ice Juice, Invoice, Choice, License

Car Carve, Scarf, Vicar, Mascara

Ref Reflex, Prefer, Careful, Barefoot

Ill Thrill, Chilly, Million, Pillow

page 41: Sentence Sleuth

1. Hawk   "Sara**h awk**wardly ..."
2. Heron   "day **her on**cologist ..."
3. Swallow "Hadrian'**s Wall, Ow**en decided..."

page 42: Give Me a Word That . . .

(Other correct answers are possible.)

1. Economical, Femininity, Justification, Magnification, Pediatrician, Perpendicular, Unbelievable
2. Ecru, Flu, Guru, Kudzu, Menu, Plateau, Tableau, Tofu, Tutu, You
3. Answer, Autumn, Ballet, Biscuit, Calf, Guess, Knee, Knife, Muscle, Sign, Sword, Wednesday, Whistle, Wrap, Yacht

page 43: Common Bonds

Theme: Bills (Dollar bills, Bill Clinton, Duck bill)

page 44: Find the Theme

Orioles, Dodgers, Pirates, Red Sox, Yankees

Theme: Baseball teams

page 45: Addables

(Other correct answers are possible.)

1. Awed, Dews, Dewy, Drew, Lewd, Owed, Wade, Weds, Weed, Weld, Wend, Wide
2. Clot, Coat, Colt, Coot, Cost, Cote, Cots, Taco, Tock
3. Chain, China, Chins, Cinch, Finch, Niche, Pinch, Winch

page 46: Do the Math!

Three days. Farmer Joe's chickens yield 60 eggs per day ($\frac{2}{3}$ x 90 = 60 chickens that lay one egg per day). Fifteen dozen = 180 eggs, divided by 60 eggs per day = three days.

page 47: Filled with Emotion

1. *Bitter*sweet
2. *Sad* sack
3. *Hate* crime
4. *Anger* management
5. Bundle of *joy*

CHAPTER TWO

page 49: Need Directions?

1. Washington, DC
2. London, England
3. The Wizard of Oz
4. Venice, Italy
5. New York City
6. New Orleans

page 50: Trimble

1. Chevrolet
2. Beetle
3. Dodge
4. France
5. Rolls-Royce

Trimble Answer: Toyota Corolla

page 52: Riddle Me This
Yes. It comes between July 3rd and July 5th.

page 53: Making Connections
Clues: Area, Zip
Theme: _____ code

Clues: Piggy, River
Theme: Types of banks

Clues: Cream, String
Theme: Types of cheese

page 54: Two by Three
(Other correct answers are possible.)
S Sunflower/Snapdragon, Saint Bernard/Shih tzu, Shingles/Stroke
A Amaryllis/Azalea, Afghan hound/Airedale terrier, AIDS/Alzheimer's
D Daisy/Dahlia, Dachshund/Dalmatian, Diabetes/Diphtheria

page 55: Secret Word: Quilting Bee
(Other correct answers are possible.)
4 Letters: Been, Beet, Belt, Bent, Bile, Bite, Blue, Bunt, Gelt, Gene, Gent, Gibe, Gilt, Glee, Glen, Glib, Glue, Glut, Lent, Lien, Lieu, Line, Lint, Lite, Lube, Luge, Lung, Lute, Nite, Quit, Teen, Tile, Tine, Tube, Tune, Unit

5 Letters: Beget, Begin, Begun, Beige, Being, Belie, Betel, Bilge, Binge, Blunt, Bugle, Built, Bulge, Elite, Genie, Guile, Guilt, Inlet, Liege, Lunge, Queen, Quiet, Quilt, Quint, Quite, Tinge, Unite, Unlit, Untie

Secret Word: Until

page 56: Say What?
1. Good fences make good neighbors.
2. Lightning never strikes in the same place twice.
3. Make hay while the sun shines.
4. See a penny, pick it up, and all day long, you'll have good luck.
5. What goes around, comes around.

page 57: One-Minute Madness: Famous People Named George
(Other correct answers are possible.)
George Burns, George Bush, George Carlin, George Clooney, George Foreman, George Gershwin, George Gobel, George Hamilton, George Harrison, George Jessel, George Lopez, George Orwell, George S. Patton, George Raft, George C. Scott, George Bernard Shaw, George Steinbrenner, George Stephanopoulos, George Wallace, George Washington, George Washington Carver

page 58: OTHER Words

1. Bathrobe
2. Earthworm
3. Orchestra
4. Thermostat
5. Ghostwriter
6. Butterscotch

page 59: Word Tower

(Other correct answers are possible.)

1. Re
2. Red
3. Rest
4. Rebel
5. Recipe
6. Recover
7. Religion
8. Rebellion

page 60: Wacky Wordy

For instance

page 61: People Rebus

1. Ringo Starr (Ring + Ghost + R)
2. Al Pacino (L + Patch + E + Nose – SE)
3. Jackie Onassis (Jack + Key + Cone – C + Glasses – GL)

page 62: What's the Word?

Fit   Profit, Fitness, Outfit, Graffiti

Lap   Lapel, Flap, Lapdog, Collapse

Rot   Trot, Rotate, Protect, Protein

Era   Erase, Opera, Camera, Ceramics

page 63: Odd Man Out

1. Pencil is the odd man out. All the rest finish the phrase "Golden _____."
2. Guitar is the odd man out. All the rest are types of chips.
3. Amendment is the odd man out. All the others finish the phrase "Old_____."
4. Cotton is the odd man out. All the rest are types of shoes.

page 64: Syllability

1. Penitentiary
   PEN • I • TEN • TIA • RY
2. Circumference
   CIR • CUM • FER • ENCE
3. Insecticide
   IN • SEC • TI • CIDE
4. Nothing
   NOTH • ING
5. Graduation
   GRAD • U • A • TION
6. Ordinary
   OR • DI • NAR • Y
7. Vocabulary
   VO • CAB • U • LAR • Y

page 66: Opposites Attract

1. Early/Late
2. Lost/Found
3. Inner/Outer
4. Circle/Line
5. Lowest/Highest

page 68: Change a Letter
(Other correct answers are possible.)
1. C: Clown, Cloud, Coup
2. C: Icon, Police, Scatter
3. G: Tiger, Goiter, Sing
4. Y: Spy, Youth, Myth

page 69: Eights & Fours
(Other correct answers are possible.)
1. Pampered   Deep/Ramp
2. Pressure   Sees/Purr

page 70: Hidden Quotation
1. Asthma, Cold, Flu, Stroke
2. Shrewd, Wise
3. Porcupine, Rat, Squirrel, Hamster
4. Yield, One way, Stop, Merge
5. Across, Near, Upon, In, Into
6. Opal, Garnet, Topaz
Quotation: Make crime pay.
Become a lawyer.

page 72: Fill In the Letters
(Other correct answers are possible.)
1. Auto, Buts, Butt, Cute, Cuts,
   Duty, Futz, Guts, Huts, Jute, Juts,
   Lute, Mute, Mutt, Nuts, Outs,
   Puts, Putt, Ruts, Tuts, Tutu
2. Asker, Baker, Biker, Faker, Hiker,
   Inker, Joker, Liker, Maker, Piker,
   Poker, Raker, Taker, Waker

page 73: Give Me a Word That . . .
(Other correct answers are possible.)

1. Beep, Bleep, Cheap, Cheep,
   Creep, Deep, Heap, Keep, Leap,
   Peep, Reap, Seep, Sheep, Steep,
   Sweep, Weep
2. Enraged, Fuming, Furious,
   Incensed, Infuriated, Irate, Livid,
   Mad, Outraged, Raging, Riled
3. Adjective, Adjourn, Adjust,
   Ajar, Banjo, Cajole, Eject, Injury,
   Major, Object, Pajamas, Project,
   Rejoice, Subject

page 74: Griddle
(Other correct answers are possible.)
4 Letters: Ante, Fair, Fare, Fear, Fife,
Fine, Fire, Floe, Font, Foul, Loft,
Loin, Near, Neon, Nine, Raft, Rain,
Rant, Rein, Rent, Rife, Riff, Rift

5 Letters: Afire, Afoul, Faint, Feint,
Finer, Fluff, Fount, Infer, Niner,
Offer, Often

6 Letters: Ireful, Refine, Teflon

7 Letters: Funnier

8 Letters: Fluffier

page 76: Order, Please!
1. 1 gallon (16 cups), 1 liter
   (4.2 cups), 3 cups
2. Hillary Clinton (1947), Elizabeth
   Warren (1949), Angela Merkel
   (1954)

page 77: Run the Alphabet: Countries

(Other correct answers are possible.)

Argentina	Netherlands
Belgium	Oman
Cambodia	Portugal
Denmark	Qatar
Egypt	Romania
Finland	Sweden
Germany	Turkey
Honduras	United States
Italy	Vietnam
Japan	W (None)
Kenya	X (None)
Laos	Yemen
Mexico	Zambia

page 78: Double Trouble

1. Home
2. Mail
3. Free
4. Trap

page 79: What's the Word?

Act Action, Cactus, Factory, Compact

Gar Garb, Cigar, Sugar, Garden

Ham Shame, Chamber, Hamlet, Hamster

Met Comet, Metro, Method, Diameter

page 80: Pictures & Letters

EYE + C	Icy
B + WITCH	Bewitch
L + BOW	Elbow
P + CAN	Pecan
N + TIRE	Entire
I + BALL	Eyeball

page 82: Memorable Movie Lines

1. Humphrey Bogart, Rick Blaine, *Casablanca* (1942)
2. Vivien Leigh, Scarlett O'Hara, *Gone With the Wind* (1939)
3. Michael Douglas, Gordon Gekko, *Wall Street* (1987)
4. Katharine Hepburn, Ethel Thayer, *On Golden Pond* (1981)
5. Richard Castellano, Clemenza, *The Godfather* (1972)

page 83: Counting Syllables

(In some cases, other correct answers are possible.)

1. Fettuccine, Macaroni, Manicotti, Orecchiette, Ravioli, Rigatoni, Tagliatelle, Tortellini, Tortelloni, Vermicelli
2. Armoire, Bookcase, Buffet, Cupboard, Daybed, Divan, Dresser, Footstool, Futon, Hassock, Headboard, Loveseat, Mattress, Nightstand, Sideboard, Sleeper, Sofa, Table, Wardrobe, Washstand, Workbench
3. Babe, Big, Dave, Doubt, Elf, Ghost, Grease, Hair, Jaws, M*A*S*H, Mask, Milk, Reds, Shrek
4. Maine

page 84: One-Minute Madness: Network and Cable TV Outlets

(Other correct answers are possible.)

A&E
ABC
AMC
Animal Planet
BBC America
BET
Bloomberg TV
Bravo
Cartoon
  Network
CBS
Cinemax
CMT
CNBC
CNN
Comedy Central
Comedy TV
Cooking
  Channel
CSPAN
Discovery
  Channel
Disney Channel
E!
ESPN
Food Network
FOX
  Broadcasting
Fox News
FX
Game Show
  Network

Hallmark
  Channel
HBO
HGTV
History
HLN
Home Shopping
  Network
IFC
Ion Television
Lifetime
Me TV
MSNBC
MTV
National
  Geographic
NBC
Nick at Nite
Nick, Jr.
Nickelodeon
Oprah Winfrey
  Network
Oxygen
PBS
Penthouse TV
Playboy TV
QVC
Showtime
Smithsonian
  Channel
Starz
Sundance TV
Syfy

TBS
Telemundo
The CW
The Weather
  Channel
TLC
TNT

Travel Channel
Turner Classic
  Movies
TV Land
Univision
USA Network
VH1

page 85: Finish the Proverb

1. *Let the punishment fit the crime.*
2. *Never put off until tomorrow what you can do today.*
3. *The best things in life are free.*
4. *You can never have too much of a good thing.*

page 86: Picture Connections

Things with keys:
Typewriter, Piano, Florida

Words that sound like a letter:
Tee, Cue, Ewe

Things with needles: Sewing machine, Phonograph, Pine tree

page 87: Presidential Quotations

1. D
2. C
3. A
4. B

page 88: Happy Endings

1. **Cal**   Vocal, Fiscal, Rascal, Logical

2. **Able** Stable, Lovable, Portable, Irritable
3. **Oon** Swoon, Baboon, Buffoon, Macaroon
4. **Tive** Native, Festive, Creative, Fugitive

page 89: It's All in the Name

1. Rob + Goo + Hurt + Lei
   Robert Goulet
2. Jewel + D + E + Annie + Rude
   Rudy Giuliani
3. Burn + Odd + Hip + Re
   Audrey Hepburn

page 90: A Potpourri of Nicknames

1. The London Metro, TV
2. Mustache
3. George W. Bush
4. The American flag
5. Amelia Earhart

page 91: Join 'Em

1. Gene R Ally   Generally
2. Memo R Able   Memorable
3. War R Ant   Warrant
4. Me R Chant   Merchant
5. Out R Age   Outrage
6. Pi R Ate   Pirate

page 92: Sentence Sleuth

1. Charleston   **"Charles to N**ana Mary. . ."
2. Disco   "husban**d is co**-editor. . ."
3. Salsa   "**is Al's** all-time . . ."

page 93: Opposites Attract

1. Wrong/Right
2. Over/Under
3. Start/Stop
4. Teach/Learn
5. Close/Open

page 94: Down to the Wire

(Other correct answers are possible.)
1. *Step up* to the plate
2. *Cut* to the chase
3. *Armed* to the teeth
4. *Hitchhiker's Guide* to the Galaxy
5. Like a *Lamb* to the slaughter

page 95: Big Boy

1. Big Blue
2. The Big Bang theory
3. The Big Dipper
4. Bigger fish to fry
5. Speak softly and carry a big stick.

page 96: Stinky Pinky

1. German sermon
2. Free brie
3. Fit Brit
4. Prune spoon
5. Best jest

page 97: FORE Words

1. Offer
2. Bonfire
3. Foreign
4. Barefoot
5. Inferior
6. Boyfriend

CHAPTER THREE

page 99: Movie Questions
1. *Field of Dreams*
2. *Dirty Harry*
3. *Taxi Driver*
4. *Ghostbusters*
5. *A Few Good Men*

page 100: Riddle Me This
She is a justice of the peace.

page 101: One-Minute Madness: Words that Mean LIE
(Other correct answers are possible.)
BS (Bullsh*t), Bull, Deceive, Deception, Dishonesty, Disinformation, Distortion, Exaggerate, Fabrication, Falsehood, Falsification, Fib, Fiction, Fudge, Hyperbole, Inaccuracy, Invention, Mendacity, Misinform, Mislead, Misrepresentation, Misspeak, Misstate, Misstatement, Myth, Perjury, Prevaricate, Propaganda, Story, Tale, Untruth, Whopper

page 102: Addables
(Other correct answers are possible.)
1. Nape, Naps, Pain, Pane, Pang, Pans, Pant, Pawn, Plan, Snap, Span
2. Digs, Ding, Gild, Gird, Grid
3. Deaf, Deft, Defy, Fade, Feed, Fend, Feud, Fled

page 103: Mathematically Speaking
1. Line
2. Pentagon
3. Plane
4. Formula
5. Parallel

page 104: Is or Isn't?
1. (c) Anthony Hopkins
2. (a) Rutgers University
3. (b) Koala
4. (a) Washington, DC

page 105: Filled with Emotion
1. *Raging* Bull
2. The Sound and the *Fury*
3. *Fear* of Flying
4. Swallow your *pride*
5. *Happy* hour

page 106: Griddle
(Other correct answers are possible.)
4 Letters
Arch, Chef, Clef, Dean, Dear, Deer, Deft, Earn, Edit, Fear, Feed, Feel, Feet, Fend, Fern, Free, Fret, Hear, Heel, Heft, Idea, Leer, Left, Near, Rand, Reed, Reef, Reel, Rend, Rhea, Teed, Teen, Tide, Tiff

5 Letters: Arced, Cheer, Cleft, Crane, Creel, Defer, Fetid, Freed, Freer, Leech, Refed, Refer, Relet

6 Letters: Arched, Craned, Credit, Defter, Differ, Feeler, Reefed, Reefer, Refeed

7 Letters: Leeched

page 108: Eights & Fours
(Other correct answers are possible.)
1. Worships   Show/Rips
2. Tapestry   Star/Type

page 109: Jingles & Slogans
1. "... my peanut butter."
   Reese's Peanut Butter Cups
2. "... to make a tender chicken."
   Perdue
3. "... Mastercard."
4. "... beef?"
   Wendy's
5. "... good men."
   US Marines

page 110: Wacky Wordy
One foot after the other

page 111: Homographs
1. Citizen
2. Cancer
3. Top
4. Trip
5. Kiwi

page 112: The Name of the Game
1. McCoy
2. Charley
3. Billy
4. Johnny
5. Alec

page 113: Making Connections
Clues: Key, Napkin
Theme: _____ ring

Clues: Check, Trampoline
Theme: Things that bounce

Clues: Income, Property
Theme: Types of taxes

page 114: Secret Word: Toothpaste
(Other correct answers are possible.)
4 Letters: Apes, Apse, Atop, East, Eats, Hasp, Hate, Hats, Heap, Heat, Hoes, Hoop, Hoot, Hope, Hops, Hose, Host, Hots, Oath, Oats, Oohs, Oops, Opts, Past, Pate, Path, Pats, Peas, Peat, Peso, Pest, Pets, Poet, Pose, Posh, Post, Pots, Sate, Seat, Shoe, Shoo, Shop, Shot, Soap, Soot, Spat, Spot, Step, Stop, Tape, Taps, Tats, Teas, Teat, Test, That, Toes, Toot, Tops, Tote, Tots

5 Letters: Ethos, Haste, Hates, Heaps, Heats, Hoops, Hoots, Hopes, Hosta, Oaths, Paste, Pates, Paths, Pesto, Phase, Photo, Poets, Shape, Shoot, Spate, State, Stoat, Stoop, Tapes, Taste, Teats, **Those** ***, Toast, Tooth, Toots, Totes

*** Secret Word

page 115: Say What?

1. The squeaky wheel gets the grease.
2. All good things must come to an end.
3. A picture is worth a thousand words.
4. Time is money.
5. Blood is thicker than water.

page 116: Word Rebus

1. Antiperspirant (Ant + Tea + Purse + Spire + Ant)
2. Neanderthal (Knee + And + Earth + Ball – B)
3. Unforgettable (Sun – S + 4 + Target – TAR + Table)

page 117: Your Highness

1. Billie Jean King
2. King Arthur
3. *The African Queen*
4. Queensland
5. The King of Swing

page 118: Scrambled States

1. Colorado
2. Oklahoma
3. Montana
4. Pennsylvania
5. North Carolina

page 119: Endings & Beginnings

1. Wise
2. Free
3. Arm
4. Radio
5. Sweet

page 120: Give Me a Word That . . .

(Other correct answers are possible.)

1. Advertise, Bachelors, Ballerina, Dissatisfaction, Grandmothers, Hospitals, Microbiology, Psychologist, Quotations, Scientific, Tangerines, Tumbleweed, Undertaker
2. Ad, As, Ax, Be, By, Do, Go, He, If, In, Is, It, Ma, Me, My, Or, Pa, So, To, Up, Us, We, Ye
3. Backbone, Backlog, Bedroom, Bookmark, Crosswalk, Eyeball, Firefighter, Fireworks, Footprint, Hometown, Honeymoon, Keyboard, Lifeguard, Moonlight, Rainbow, Skateboard, Sunflower, Toothpaste, Update

page 121: What's the Word?

Don Donate, Abandon, Donkey, Tendon

Out Outside, Mouth, Boutique, Devout

Win Dwindle, Window, Snowing, Twinkle

For Afford, Comfort, Forbid, Before

page 122: Run the Alphabet: Companies

(Other correct answers are possible.)

Allstate	Nike
Bloomingdale's	Old Navy
Coca-Cola	Perdue
Disney	Quality Inn
Exxon Mobil	Raytheon
FedEx	Samsung
Goodyear	Target
Harley-Davidson	UPS
IBM	Volvo
J. C. Penney	Whole Foods
Kellogg's	Xerox
Lowe's	Yahoo!
McDonald's	Zale's

page 123: Word Tower

(Other correct answers are possible.)

1. To
2. Top
3. Tofu
4. Toast
5. Toffee
6. Tobacco

7. Together
8. Toothache

page 124: Odd Man Out

1. *Nose* is the odd man out. You have only one of those. All the rest come in pairs.

2. *North* is the odd man out. Oliver North was involved in the Iran-Contra scandal. All the others are last names of people involved in the Watergate scandal.

3. *Turk* is the old man out. All the rest finish the phrase "Great _____ ."

4. *Chariots of Fire* is the odd man out. All the other films are set (in whole or in part) in Ireland/Northern Ireland.

page 125: Change a Letter

(Other correct answers are possible.)

1. H: The, Hinge, Phone
2. R: Irk, Ratio, Prayer
3. W: Knew, Wager, Newer
4. P: Chapter, Slop, Pallet

page 126: Letter Play

1. Count
2. Danger
3. Grant
4. Party
5. Tack
6. Cried
7. Lamb

Letter Play Word: Bargain

page 127: Opposites Attract

1. Won/Lost
2. Open/Shut
3. Lives/Dies
4. Save/Spend
5. Best/Worst

page 128: Hidden Quotation

1. Eat, Under, Arson, Ink, Over
2. Bush
3. Nip/Pin, Stop/Pots, Devil/Lived, May/Yam
4. Butter, Giraffe, Fluffy
5. Mania, Radio, Video
6. Venus, Mars, Jupiter

Quotation: You will become the person you decide to be.

page 130: Do the Math!

6 hours and 10 minutes
(1:17 + 1:46 + 3:07)

page 132: FOOL Words

1. Follow
2. Forlorn
3. Spoonful
4. Foxhole
5. Falsehood
6. Childproof

page 133: Is or Isn't?

1. (c) Mezquita (which is the Spanish word for *mosque*)
2. (b) Cimarron
3. (d) Shark
4. (c) Pentagon

page 134: One-Minute Madness: San or Santa Cities

(Other correct answers are possible.)

San Angelo, San Antonio, San Bernardino, San Clemente, San Diego, San Francisco, San Jose, San Juan Capistrano, San Luis Obispo, San Mateo, San Rafael, Santa Anita, Santa Anna, Santa Barbara, Santa Clara, Santa Cruz, Santa Fe, Santa Monica, Santa Rosa

page 135: Animal Watching

A. Aardvark
B. Possum
C. Porcupine
D. Armadillo

page 136: A Pair of Riddles

1. Anything. Buildings don't jump.
2. A palm

page 137: Double Trouble

1. Room
2. Pocket
3. Fight
4. Dollar

page 138: Wacky Wordy

That's beside the point

page 139: ColorFill

1. *Red* light district
2. *Yellow* journalism
3. Talk a *blue* streak
4. *Purple* heart

page 140: Picture Connections

Types of beans: String, Pinto, Navy

The number 3: Three o'clock, Three Little Pigs, Three-prong plug

Companies/Stores: Staples, Target, Apple

page 141: Counting Syllables

(Other correct answers are possible.)

1. Chintz, Crepe, Felt, Flax, Fleece, Gauze, Hemp, Jute, Knit, Lace, Mesh, Silk, Voile, Wool
2. Acura, Cadillac, Chevrolet, De Soto, Ferrari, Isuzu, Land Rover, Mercury, Oldsmobile, Pontiac, Subaru, Suzuki, Toyota, Volkswagen
3. Bass, Bat, Bear, Bee, Cat, Cod, Cow, Crab, Crow, Deer, Dog, Dove, Duck, Eel, Elk, Fish, Flea, Fly, Fox, Frog, Goat, Goose, Hawk, Horse, Loon, Lynx, Mink, Moose, Mouse, Mule, Ox, Pig, Rat, Shark, Sheep, Shrimp, Skunk, Sloth, Snake, Squid, Stork, Swan, Wolf
4. Austin, Boston, Charlotte, Cleveland, Dallas, Denver, Detroit, Fort Worth, Houston, Memphis, Nashville, New York, Oakland, Phoenix, Portland, Richmond, Tampa, Tucson, Tulsa

page 142: Finish the Proverb

1. *A friend in need is a* friend indeed.
2. *As snug as a bug in* a rug.
3. *Into each life a little rain* must fall.
4. *It's always darkest before* the dawn.

page 143: Sentence Sleuth

1. Apple "wire**tap ple**dges . . ."
2. Tangerine "Mus**tang, Erin e**scaped"
3. Lemon "availab**le Mon**days . . ."

page 144: Seeing Stars

1. Lone Star State
2. Star of David
3. "The Star-Spangled Banner"
4. "Stardust"
5. Star-crossed

page 145: Common Bonds

Theme: Parts of a computer
(Mouse, Screen, Keys)

page 146: Fill In the Letters

(Other correct answers are possible.)

1. Birds, Cards, Cords, Hardy, Horde, Lords, Nerdy, Tardy, Wards, Words, Wordy, Yards
2. Aide, Aids, Bide, Bids, Hide, Kids, Lids, Ride, Rids, Side, Tide, Tidy, Wide

page 147: Order, Please!

1. One large hard-boiled egg (78 calories), One medium banana (105 calories), One cup of peas (125 calories)
2. Nevada (110,570 square miles), Washington (71,300 square miles), New York (54,500 square miles)

CHAPTER FOUR

page 149: Stinky Pinky

1. Weak Greek
2. Clean queen
3. Cheese keys
4. Havana banana
5. Salad ballad

page 150: Addables

(Other correct answers are possible.)

1. Abuts, Bouts, Bunts, Burst, Busts, Busty, Butts, Stubs, Tubas, Tubes
2. Bring, Grain, Grind, Grins, Groin, Reign, Rings, Ruing, Wring
3. Cheer, Ether, Sheer, There, Three, Where

page 151: Secret Word: Fried Fish

(Other correct answers are possible.)

4 Letters: Dies, Dire, Dish, Fife, Fire, Firs, Fish, Heir, Herd, Hers, Hide, Hire, Ides, Iris, Reds, Refs, Ride, Rids, Rife, **Riff *****, Rise, Serf, Shed, Side, Sire

5 Letters: Dries, Fifed, Fifer, Fifes, Fired, Fires, Fresh, Fried, Fries, Heirs, Herds, Hides, Hired, Hires, Rides, Riffs, Serif, Shied, Shire, Shred, Sired

*** Secret Word

page 152: Acronym Alphabet

1. Bavarian Motor Works (Bayerische Motoren Werke)
2. Federal Communications Commission
3. Mobile Army Surgical Hospital
4. Video cassette recorder
5. Cardio-pulmonary resuscitation
6. Reserve Officer Training Corps

page 153: People Rebus

1. Alexander Hamilton (L + X + Hand – H + Fur – F + Ham + Pill – P + Ton)
2. Ruby Dee (Ruler – LER + Bee + D)
3. Frankenstein (Frank + N + Stein)

page 154: Word Tower
(Other correct answers are possible.)
1. Al
2. Ale
3. Also
4. Alley
5. Alarms
6. Allergy
7. Although
8. Alligator

page 155: Eights & Fours
(Other correct answers are possible.)
1. Lemonade   Meal/Done
2. Platform   Flop/Mart

page 156: Give Me a Word That . . .
(In most cases, other correct answers are possible.)
1. Accent, Announce, Bitter, Bubble, Caddy, Dilemma, Eggs, Good, Happy, Hissing, Offer, Parallel, Pizza, Quill, Sleeve, Terror, Vacuum
2. Absorb, Adverb, Bathtub, Blab, Cherub, Comb, Crumb, Disturb, Flashbulb, Grub, Knob, Nightclub, Proverb, Scab, Scrub, Snob, Thumb, Verb
3. All

page 157: One-Minute Madness: Baseball Positions
Batter, Catcher, Center field, First base, First-base coach, First-base umpire, Home-plate umpire, Left field, Left-field umpire, Pinch hitter, Pitcher, Right field, Right-field umpire, Second base, Second-base umpire, Shortstop, Third base, Third-base coach, Third-base umpire

page 158: Two by Three
(Other correct answers are possible.)
C   Cricket/Cicada, Chosen/Cookie, Charleston/Cheyenne

A   Ant/Aphid, Always/Afford, Austin/Albany

B   Bedbug/Butterfly, Beauty/Bright, Boston/Berkeley

page 159: Say What?
1. Out of sight, out of mind.
2. There is no such thing as a free lunch.
3. If you want something done right, do it yourself.
4. Talk until you are blue in the face.
5. That's the way the cookie crumbles.

page 160: Syllability
1. Genesis
   GEN • E • SIS
2. Television
   TEL • E • VI • SION
3. Envelope
   EN • VEL • OPE

4. Avocado
   AV • O • CA • DO
5. Cookie
   COOK • IE
6. Condominium
   CON • DO • MIN • I • UM
7. Dinosaurs
   DI • NO • SAURS
8. Apologize
   A • POL • O • GIZE

page 162: Griddle

(Other correct answers are possible.)
4 Letters: Ales, Arts, Arty, Bear, Bets, Blot, Blue, Boys, Buss, Busy, Byes, Byte, Easy, Eras, Lass, Leas, Less, Lets, Lobe, Lobs, Lost, Lots, Lube, Lyre, Obey, Oral, Ores, Orts, Real, Roes, Ryes, Sale, Seal, Sear, Sets, Sobs, Sole, Subs, Teal, Tear, Teas, Toys, Trey, User, Year, Yeas

5 Letters: Alert, Artsy, Beryl, Blots, Bolus, Bytes, Class, Clear, Laser, Lobes, Lubes, Lyres, Obeys, Orals, Rebel, Rebus, Seals, Sober, Steal, Stole, Style, Teals, Teary, Tress, Treys

6 Letters: Alerts, Claret, Oyster, Sclera, Steals, Stress, Stylus, Subset, Treble

7 Letters: Clarets, Subsets

page 164: Opposites Attract

1. Fat/Thin
2. First/Last
3. Past/Present
4. Deep/Shallow
5. Small/Large

page 166: Hidden Quotation

1. Japan, Iran, India, Oman
2. Alley (Kirstie), Long (Shelley), Wendt (George), Danson (Ted)
3. Grumpy, Dopey, Doc
4. Business, Believe, Stitches, Grateful
5. Labor, Energy, State
6. Mile, Cup, Yard

Quotation: If you're going through hell, keep going.

page 168: Happy Endings

1. **Rous** Porous, Generous, Numerous, Vigorous
2. **Ugh** Laugh, Enough, Through, Hiccough
3. **Ult** Vault, Occult, Result, Assault
4. **Ign** Reign, Assign, Foreign, Campaign

page 169: Riddle Me This

Twelve

page 170: Making Connections

Clues: HUD, DOJ
Theme: Federal agencies

Clues: 3^2, IX
Theme: Equals 9

Clues: Sat, Wed
Theme: Days of the week

page 171: Join 'Em
1. Eye L Ash   Eyelash
2. Too L Box   Toolbox
3. So L Id   Solid
4. Know L Edge   Knowledge
5. Imp L Ore   Implore
6. Shoe L Aces   Shoelaces

page 172: Don't . . . What?
(Other correct answers are possible.)
1. Don't ask, don't tell.
2. Don't bite off more than you can chew.
3. Don't bite the hand that feeds you.
4. Don't burn the candle at both ends.
5. Don't change horses in midstream.
6. Don't count your chickens before they hatch.
7. Don't cross a bridge before you come to it.
8. Don't cut off your nose to spite your face.
9. Don't fence me in.
10. Don't give up the ship.
11. Don't judge a book by its cover.
12. Don't look a gift horse in the mouth.
13. Don't make a mountain out of a molehill.
14. Don't play with fire.
15. Don't put all your eggs in one basket.
16. Don't put off till tomorrow what you can do today.
17. Don't put the cart before the horse.
18. Don't rain on my parade.
19. Don't take any wooden nickels.
20. Don't throw good money after bad.
21. Don't throw the baby out with the bathwater.

page 173: Dog Eat Dog
1. In the doghouse
2. Raining cats and dogs
3. Every dog has its day
4. Let sleeping dogs lie
5. Mad dogs and Englishmen

page 174: Letter Play
1. Candle
2. Player
3. Ears
4. Purse
5. Explode
6. Globe
7. Perch
8. Mister
Letter Play Word: Decibels

page 175: Word Rebus

1. Cubicle (Cube + Pickle – P)
2. Museum (Music – IC + Z + Drum – DR)
3. Apologetic (Apple – PLE + Paw + Halo – HA + Jet + Tick)

page 176: It's Time!

1. 14
2. 1,000
3. 1,200 (12 x 100)
4. 87 (4 x 20 + 7)

page 177: Change a Letter

1. V: Avid, Invite, Leave
2. L: Butler, Drivel, Filled
3. O: Oat, Bingo, Bottle
4. L: Owls, Caller, Scalp

page 178: It's All in the Name

1. Key + Crews + Ta + Nick + Chef
   Nikita Khrushchev
2. Don + Sun + John + Lynde
   Lyndon Johnson
3. Ah + Bench + Mince + Spock
   Benjamin Spock

page 179: Double Trouble

1. Worm
2. Crow
3. Wolf
4. Turkey
5. Chicken

page 180: Identify This!

1. Scottish fold
2. Balaclava
3. Kinkajou
4. Spork
5. Geoduck
6. F-hole

page 182: FLAG Words

1. Frugal
2. Fragile
3. Leapfrog
4. Grateful
5. Floodgate
6. Lifeguard

page 183: Riddle Me This

February. It's the shortest month of the year.

page 184: Odd Man Out

1. *Cormorant* is the odd man out. It is a bird. All the others are constellations.
2. *Shuttlecock* is the odd man out. It is the cone-shaped object you bat in badminton. All the rest are characters from Shakespeare.
3. *Quiche* is the odd man out. It is an egg-and-cheese pie. All the others are soups.
4. *Gettysburg* is the odd man out. It is located in Pennsylvania. All the rest are located in New York.

page 185: Saintly Things

1. St. Joseph
2. St. Jude
3. St. Elsewhere
4. *The Spirit of St. Louis*
5. St. John's wort
6. The Church of Jesus Christ of Latter-Day Saints

page 186: Presidential Quotations

1. D
2. A
3. C
4. B

page 187: Word Tower

(Other correct answers are possible.)

1. Ta
2. Tab
3. Tack
4. Tally
5. Target
6. Tabloid
7. Taxpayer
8. Tangerine

page 188: Opposites Attract

1. Rested/Tired
2. Fast/Slow
3. Love/Hate
4. Angel/Devil
5. Break/Repair

page 190: What's the Word?

Oil Boil, Spoil, Toilet, Turmoil
Sue Issue, Tissue, Suede, Pursue
Tic Tick, Stick, Ticket, Frantic
Van Divan, Vanity, Advance, Vanilla

page 191: Eights & Fours

(Other correct answers are possible.)

| 1. | Wardrobe | Wore/Drab |
| 2. | Baseball | Able/Labs |

page 192: Picture Connections

Types of knives: Steak, Jack, Butter

Things with strings: Apron, Guitar, Kite

Things with trunks: Tree, Auto, Elephant

page 193: Give Me a Word That . . .

(Other correct answers are possible.)

1. Acquaintance, Acquire, Antique, Aquarium, Burlesque, Conquer, Critique, Delinquent, Eloquent, Equal, Equator, Frequent, Headquarters, Liquid, Mosque, Opaque, Sequins, Squad, Square, Squint
2. Black, Clock, Cross, Dress, Month, Plant, Right, Smart, Spank, Start, Storm, Thing, Think, Watch, Witch, World

3. Ailing, Feeling poorly, Frail, Ill, In a bad way, In poor health, Indisposed, Off, On medication, Queasy, Suffering, Under the weather, Unhealthy, Unwell

page 194: One-Minute Madness: _____ Water

(Other correct answers are possible.)
Backwater, Bath water, Bottled water, Carbonated water, Cold water, Deep water, Dishwater, Distilled water, Firewater, Floodwater, Fresh water, Groundwater, Hard water, Holy water, Hot water, Ice water, Make water, Mineral water, Open water, Pass water, Purified water, Rainwater, Rose water, Rough water, Salt water, Seawater, Seltzer water, Sewer water, Soda water, Sparkling water, Spring water, Still water, Sugar water, Tap water, Toilet water, Tonic water, Tread water, Underwater, Wastewater, Well water, White water

page 195: Jingles & Slogans

1. "... maybe it's Maybelline."
2. "... picker-upper."
   Bounty paper towels
3. "... Sara Lee."
4. "... a Klondike Bar?"
5. "... got the beer."
   Miller High Life

page 196: Pictures & Parts

Coo + KEY	Cookie
SAW + Sage	Sausage
CASH + Ew	Cashew
GUM + Bo	Gumbo
Brow + KNEES	Brownies
Arti + CHOKE	Artichoke

CHAPTER FIVE

page 199: Is or Isn't?

1. (c) Rabbit (Volkswagen)
2. (b) Brownie Bits
3. (b) Provincetown
4. (b) To everything there is a season.

page 200: Wacky Wordy

Unfinished Symphony

page 201: Two by Three

(Other correct answers are possible.)
H   Hunt/Hope, Hazel/Hot pink, Haiti/Honduras
I   Ink/Inch, Indigo/Ivory, Israel/Iceland
T   Thought/Them, Teal/Turquoise, Turkey/Taiwan

page 202: Common Bonds

Theme: Honey _____
(Honeycomb, Honeymoon, Honeybee)

page 203: Endings & Beginnings
1. Tail
2. Dog
3. Face
4. Travel
5. Nail

page 204: Secret Word: Idaho Potato
(Other correct answers are possible.)
4 Letters: Atop, Data, Doth, Hood, Hoop, Hoot, Iota, Oath, Paid, Path, Pita, Pith, Pooh, **That *****, Toad, Toot

5 Letters: Adapt, Adopt, Aphid, Ditto, Patio, Photo, Tooth

*** Secret Word

page 205: Mathematically Speaking
1. Square
2. Circle
3. Cube
4. Proof
5. Triangle

page 206: Hidden Quotation
1. Knife, Psalm, Aisle, Writer
2. Water, Soda, Juice
3. Bicycle, Bus
4. Level, Libel, Legal

5. C, IX, M
6. Touch, Taste
Quotation: Whatever you are, be a good one.

page 208: Stinky Pinky
1. Norway doorway
2. Felon melon
3. Mobster lobster
4. Gazelle hotel
5. Fish's dishes

page 209: Join 'Em
1. Cap T Ion   Caption
2. Fox T Rot   Foxtrot
3. Hear T Burn   Heartburn
4. Gems T One   Gemstone
5. Boom T Own   Boomtown
6. Pain T Brush   Paintbrush

page 210: Run the Alphabet: Ends in O
(Other correct answers are possible.)

Armadillo	No
Banjo	Oregano
Cello	Piano
Disco	Quarto
Echo	Radio
Flamingo	Shampoo
Gazebo	Tornado
Hero	Undo
Into	Vertigo
Jumbo	Weirdo
Kimono	X *(None)*
Logo	Yoyo
Mango	Zoo

page 211: Geographical Nicknames

1. Atlanta
2. Beijing
3. Chicago
4. Salem (Massachusetts)
5. Honolulu

page 212: You Can't . . . What?

(Other correct answers are possible.)

1. You can't teach an old dog new tricks.
2. You can't win 'em all.
3. You can't always get what you want.
4. You can't get there from here.
5. You can't go home again.
6. You can't have your cake and eat it too.
7. You can't hurry love.
8. You can't judge a book by its cover.
9. You can't live on bread alone.
10. You can't make a silk purse out of a sow's ear.
11. You can't make an omelet without breaking a few eggs.
12. You can't see the forest for the trees.
13. You can't squeeze blood out of a stone.
14. You can't take it with you.
15. You can't unscramble a scrambled egg.
16. You can't wake a person who is pretending to be asleep.

page 213: Sentence Sleuth

1. Waltz   "**Walt, z**ip . . ."
2. Limbo "to c**limb o**ver. . ."
3. Ballet   "basket**ball, et**c."

page 214: Number Words

1. Be4   Before or Be9   Benign
2. Sk8   Skate
3. 2th   Tooth
4. 4k   Fork
5. Ba6   Basics

page 215: One-Minute Madness: Occupations Beginning with S

(Other correct answers are possible.)

Salesperson, School bus driver, School counselor, School librarian, School nurse, School principal, School psychologist, Scientist, Screenwriter, Scuba diver, Sculptor, Secretary, Secretary of state, Security guard, Seismologist, Senator, Sheriff, Shipbuilder, Short-order cook, Sign language interpreter, Singer, Social worker, Sociologist, Soldier, Sound recordist, Special agent, Special education teacher, Speech-language pathologist, Sports agent, Sportscaster, Stage manager, Stained glass artist, Statistician, Stenographer, Still photographer, Stockbroker, Stonemason, Streetcar operator, Stripper, Structural engineer, Surgeon, Surgeon general, Surveyor, Switchboard operator

page 216: CODE Words

1. Comedy
2. Second
3. Condemn
4. Chowder
5. Education
6. Announced

page 217: Word Tower

(Other correct answers are possible.)

1. Ha
2. Ham
3. Halt
4. Hasty
5. Hazard
6. Harmony
7. Handsome
8. Happiness

page 218: Say What?

1. Don't cut off your nose to spite your face.
2. An ounce of prevention is worth a pound of cure.
3. Diamonds are a girl's best friend.
4. Put your money where your mouth is.
5. The best thing since sliced bread.

page 219: Addables

(Other correct answers are possible.)

1. Airs, Bris, Firs, Iris, Irks, Ribs, Rids, Rigs, Rims, Rips, Rise, Risk, Sari, Sire, Sirs, Stir

2. Aunt, Bunt, Hunt, Nuts, Punt, Runt, Stun, Tuna, Tune, Turn, Unit, Unto
3. Ached, Aches, Beach, Cache, Chafe, Chase, Cheap, Cheat, Leach, Peach, Reach, Teach

page 220: Griddle

(Other correct answers are possible.)

4 Letters: Aria, Arid, Dart, Daze, Dolt, Doze, Dram, Earl, Liar, Lira, Lord, Maid, Mail, Mart, Maze, Mild, Raid, Rail, Raze, Tail, Tram, Trim, Trod, Wear, Weir, Word, Writ

5 Letters: Amaze, Atria, Drama, Maize, Raita, Razor, Trail, Triad, Weird, World

6 Letters: Lizard, Tailor

7 Letters: Airmail

9 Letters: Dramatize

page 222: Happy Endings

1. **Ple** Apple, Maple, Simple, Steeple
2. **Orm** Storm, Inform, Conform, Uniform
3. **Itch** Pitch, Switch, Twitch, Bewitch
4. **Lly** Bully, Woolly, Finally, Casually

page 223: Word Rebus

1. Accelerate (Ax + L + Meter – MET + 8)
2. Adolescence (Plaid – PL + Doll + S + Cents)
3. Absolutely (Abs + Sew + Lute + Leaf – F)

page 224: Give Me a Word That . . .

(Other correct answers are possible.)

1. Bonjour (French), Hola (Spanish), Hallo/Guten Tag (German), Ciao (Italian), Konichiwa (Japanese), Marhabaan (Arabic), Ni hao (Chinese), Aloha (Hawaiian), Shalom (Hebrew), Olá (Portuguese)
2. Ace, Adieu, Age, Aioli, Area, Auk, Bee, Boa, Eave, Eerie, Fee, Idea, Oak, Oleo, Ooze, Owe, Queue
3. Bill, Bolt, Charge, Clip, Club, Crane, Date, Draft, Glass, Grand, Jam, Leaves, Mine, Mint, Pound, Prune, Right, Rose, Season, Yard

page 225: Odd Man Out

1. *Either* is the odd man out. It is a conjunction. All the other words are prepositions.
2. *Eisenhower* is the odd man out. All the others were US vice presidents who never became president.

3. *Cyprus* is the odd man out. It is located in the Mediterranean. All the rest are islands in the Caribbean.
4. *The Big Sleep* is the odd man out. All the rest are films starring Katharine Hepburn.

page 226: Eights & Fours

(Other correct answers are possible.)

1. Gangster   Gets/Rang
2. Daydream   Dead/Army

page 227: Letter Play

1. Lust
2. Sly
3. Stable
4. Calmer
5. Does
6. Right

Letter Play Word: Rumble

page 229: Making Connections

Clues: BS, JD
Theme: College or graduate degrees

Clues: PI, MU
Theme: Greek letters

Clues: MI, VI
Theme: Roman numerals
(MI = 1,001, VI = 6)

page 230: Syllability

1. Academic
   AC • A • DEM • IC

2. Cannibal
   CAN • NI • BAL
3. Delinquent
   DE • LIN • QUENT
4. Produce
   PRO • DUCE
5. Vivid
   VIV • ID
6. Injection
   IN • JEC • TION
7. Horrible
   HOR • RI • BLE
8. Merchandise
   MER • CHAN • DISE
9. Dermatology
   DER • MA • TOL • O • GY

page 232: Scrambled States
1. New Hampshire
2. Alabama
3. Maryland
4. Michigan
5. South Carolina

page 233: Opposites Attract
1. East/West
2. Attic/Cellar
3. Begin/End
4. Cruel/Kind
5. Friend/Enemy

page 234: Two by Three
(Other correct answers are possible.)
G Geologist/Governor, Gall
   bladder/Gums, Goose/Goldfinch

E Engineer/Electrician, Eye/
   Esophagus, Eagle/Egret
M Mailman/Magician, Molars/
   Muscles, Magpie/Mockingbird

page 235: Change a Letter
1. U: Value, Umpire, Revenue
2. S: Post, Whistle, Quarts
3. O: Too, Who, Soar
4. B: Brine, Lamb, Cubed

page 236: Picture Titles
Rear Window
Midnight Cowboy
Treasure Island

page 237: Order, Please!
1. Podiatrist $150,000, Pharmacist
   $126,000, Nurse practitioner
   $105,000
2. Tennessee Ave. (Orange) $60,
   Indiana Ave. (Red) $220, Marvin
   Gardens (Yellow) $280

page 238: KIND Words
1. Kidney
2. Duckling
3. Wrinkled
4. Quicksand
5. Candlestick
6. Windbreaker

page 239: Sentence Sleuth
1. France "Cliff **ran** **Ce**ntral City..."
2. Chile "hiba**chi**," **Le**ster said...
3. Panama "one **pan, a Ma**ytag..."

page 240: Riddle Me This

Friday is his horse's name.

page 241: It's All in the Name

1. Anne + L + Mark + Meg
   Meghan Markle
2. Mare + E + Clue + Rows + Knee
   Rosemary Clooney
3. Ron + James + Lab
   LeBron James

page 242: Run the Alphabet: TV Shows

(Many other correct answers are possible.)

All My Children	*NYPD Blue*
Bonanza	*The Odd Couple*
Candid Camera	*Perry Mason*
Downton Abbey	*Queen for a Day*
Ed Sullivan Show	*Roseanne*
Family Feud	*Seinfeld*
Get Smart	*Taxi*
Hawaii Five-O	*Ugly Betty*
I've Got a Secret	*Vega$*
The Jetsons	*What's My Line?*
Knots Landing	*The X-Files*
L.A. Law	*You Bet Your Life*
M*A*S*H	*Zorro*

page 243: Picture Connections

Shoe parts: Lace, Heel, Tongue

Baseball terms: Swing, Strike, Fly

Keyboard keys: Escape, Shift, Tab

page 244: Double Trouble

1. Law
2. Name
3. Grand
4. White

page 245: Need Directions?

1. Tokyo, Japan
2. Memphis, TN
3. San Francisco, CA
4. In the funny pages
5. Pakistan (near Afghanistan)
6. Jerusalem

page 246: What's the Word?

The Theory, Atheist, Breathe, Clothes

Ski Skip, Skill, Asking, Pigskin

Ram Tramp, Framed, Ramble, Ceramic

Lie Flies, Alien, Goalie, Relief

page 247: Ted's Terrible Titles

1. *From Here to Eternity*
   (James Jones)
2. *Tender Is the Night*
   (F. Scott Fitzgerald)
3. *Pride and Prejudice*
   (Jane Austen)
4. *The Call of the Wild*
   (Jack London)
5. *Crime and Punishment*
   (Fyodor Dostoevsky)
6. *White Fang*
   (Jack London)

CHAPTER SIX

page 249: Give Me a Word That . . .
(In most cases, other correct answers are possible.)
1. Knead, Knee, Kneel, Knickers, Knife, Knight, Knit, Knob, Knock, Knockwurst, Knot, Know, Knowledge, Knuckles
2. Buzzed, Crocked, Feeling no pain, High, Inebriated, Lit, Plastered, Sloshed, Stewed, Stoned, Three sheets to the wind, Tight, Tipsy, Under the influence, Under the table, Wasted
3. Canoe

page 250: Hidden Quotation
1. Cat, Raccoon, Owl
2. Norman, Andrew
3. Rivers, Baez, Crawford
4. Triangle, Lunatic, Canopy
5. Nova, Camry, Dart
6. Level, Madam, Kayak

Quotation: A person who never made a mistake never tried anything new.

page 252: Find the Theme
Starz, Fox News, Lifetime, Bravo, ESPN
Theme: Cable TV outlets

page 253: One-Minute Madness: Caribbean Islands
(Other correct answers are possible.)
Anguilla, Antigua and Barbuda, Aruba, Bahamas, Barbados, British Virgin Islands, Cayman Islands, Cuba, Curaçao, Dominica, Grenada, Guadeloupe, Jamaica, Martinique, Montserrat, Puerto Rico, Saint Barthelemy, Saint Kitts and Nevis, Saint Lucia, Saint Martin/Saint Maarten, Trinidad and Tobago, Turks and Caicos, US Virgin Islands

page 254: Counting Syllables
(In some cases, other correct answers are possible.)
1. Castanets, Clarinet, Dulcimer, Harpsichord, Mandolin, Piccolo, Recorder, Saxophone, Tambourine, Triangle, Viola, Violin, Xylophone
2. Alpha-bits, Cheerios, Cocoa Puffs, Cream of Wheat, Frosted Flakes, Granola, Lucky Charms, Quaker Oats, Raisin Bran, Rice Krispies, Shredded Wheat, Special K,
3. Chad, France, Greece, Spain
4. January, February

page 255: One-Minute Madness: Cookies

(Other correct answers are possible.)
Animal crackers, Arrowroot Biscuits, Biscoff, Biscotti, Black-and-white cookies, Chips Ahoy, Chocolate chip cookies, Danish butter cookies, Famous Amos, Fig Newtons, Florentines, Fortune cookies, Ginger snaps, Graham crackers, Hydrox, Keebler Chips Deluxe, Lorna Doone, Macarons, Madeleines, Milano, Mint Milano, Mrs. Fields, Oatmeal cookies, Oreo, Peanut butter cookies, Pecan Sandies, Refrigerator cookies, Samoas, Sugar cookies, Sugar wafers, Tagalongs, Thin Mints, Toll House cookies, Vanilla Wafers, Vienna Fingers

page 256: People Rebus

1. Coretta Scott King (Core + Cigarette – Ciga + Bus – B + Cot + King)
2. Tchaikovsky (China – NA + Coffee – EE + Ski)
3. Tennessee Ernie Ford (10 + S + C + Fern – F + Knee + Ford)

page 258: Say What?

1. Don't bite the hand that feeds you.
2. Honesty is the best policy.
3. Hope for the best, prepare for the worst.
4. No sooner said than done.
5. You can lead a horse to water, but you can't make him drink.

page 259: Word Tower

(Other correct answers are possible.)
1. We
2. Wet
3. Weld
4. Weird
5. Weekly
6. Welcome
7. Weekends
8. Wealthier

page 260: Odd Man Out

1. *Garage* is the odd man out. All the others are types of sticks.
2. *Wishbone* is the odd man out. It is a chicken bone. All the rest are types of smoking pipes.
3. *Paris* is the odd man out. All the rest are types of apples.
4. *Bolivia* is the odd man out. It is in South America. All the other countries are in Central America.

page 261: Eights & Fours

(Other correct answers are possible.)
1. Daughter   Hate/Drug
2. Favorite   Fair/Vote

page 262: Pictures & Parts

Pion + EAR	Pioneer
PLANET + Arium	Planetarium
Intro + DEUCE	Introduce
Astro + KNOT	Astronaut
Con + TENT	Content
ANT + Enna	Antenna

page 264: Hidden Quotation

1. Desk, Sofa
2. May, Blair, Thatcher
3. Butter, Lemon, Corn, Banana
4. Mile, Yard, Meter, Inch
5. Mirror, Lightbulb, Window

Quotation: I like children, if they are properly cooked.

page 266: Join 'Em

1.	Bomb	S	Hell	Bombshell
2.	Cork	S	Crew	Corkscrew
3.	Dome	S	Tic	Domestic
4.	Eye	S	Ore	Eyesore
5.	Go	S	Sip	Gossip
6.	Him	S	Elf	Himself

page 267: ColorFill

1. *Golden* parachute
2. *Pink* panther/*Black* Panther
3. Agent *Orange*
4. *Yellow* submarine

page 268: There's No . . . What?

(Other correct answers are possible.)

1. There's no accounting for taste.
2. There's no business like show business.
3. There's no "I" in team.
4. There's no peace for the wicked.
5. There's no place like home.
6. There's no rest for the weary.
7. There's no such thing as a free lunch.
8. There's no such thing as bad publicity.
9. There's no time like the present.
10. There's no fool like an old fool.

page 269: Do the Math!
(Smallest number to largest)

2/6   1/2   5/8 (The lowest common denominator is 24.
8/24   12/24   15/24)

16/8   13/4   9/2 (Convert each improper fraction to a compound fraction.
16/8 = 2, 13/4=3 1/4, and
9/2 = 4 1/2)

.1 is the same as .10. When you add the zero, it then becomes obvious that the order from smallest to largest is .05, .10, .15, and .75. You can also think about this as fractions of a dollar, or pennies.

B	Y		T	H	E		T	I	M	E		Y	O	U	'
R	E		E	I	G	H	T	Y		Y	E	A	R	S	
O	L	D		Y	O	U	'	V	E		L	E	A	R	N
E	D		E	V	E	R	Y	T	H	I	N	G	.		
Y	O	U		O	N	L	Y		H	A	V	E		T	O
	R	E	M	E	M	B	E	R		I	T	.			

By the time you're eighty years old you've learned everything. You only have to remember it.

page 271: Who's Asking?

1. Senator Howard Baker (during the Watergate hearings)
2. Simon & Garfunkel
3. Peggy Lee
4. Katie Couric (to vice presidential candidate Sarah Palin)
5. Attorney Joseph Welch, acting as Special Counsel for the US Army. (Welch put this question to soon-to-be-disgraced Wisconsin senator Joseph McCarthy.)

page 272: Change a Letter

(Other correct answers are possible.)
1. A: Way, Saga, Broad
2. X: Fix, Coax, Exit
3. I: Waited, Failed, Irate
4. P: Accept, Compute, Spite

page 273: Riddle Me This

David

page 274: Double Trouble

1. Tax
2. Road
3. Money
4. English

page 275: Sentence Sleuth

1. Banana "tu**ba**," **Na**na told . . ."
2. Papaya "Grand**pa, Pay a** little. . ."
3. Pomegranate "Gesta**po, Meg ran a te**ach-in. . ."

page 276: Word Rebus

1. Audience (Paw – P + D + Fence – F)
2. Minorities (Miner – ER + Oar + Mitt – M + Tees)
3. Anonymity (Can – C + Pawn – P + Swim – SW + Knit – KN + T)

page 277: Whose Biography?

1. Ernest Hemingway
2. Maya Angelou

3. Anthony Bourdain
4. Nelson Mandela
5. Ernesto "Che" Guevara

page 278: Endings & Beginnings
1. Paper
2. Food
3. Ghost
4. Mine
5. Record

page 279: Say What?
1. I'll cross that bridge when I come to it.
2. You can't fool all the people all the time.
3. See you later, alligator.
4. Time flies when you're having fun.
5. If you can't beat 'em, join 'em.

page 280: Letter Play
1. Pole
2. Pamper
3. Quit
4. Parted
5. These
Letter Play Word: Storm

page 281: Filled with Emotion
1. Green with *envy*
2. Buyer's *remorse*
3. *Glee* Club
4. Taken by *surprise*
5. More's the *pity*

page 282: Fill In the Letters
(Other correct answers are possible.)
1. Dead, Deed, Died, Dyad, Dyed
2. Bandy, Candy, Canny, Dandy, Fancy, Fanny, Handy, Hanky, Lanky, Mangy, Manly, Nanny, Pansy, Panty, Randy, Rangy, Sandy, Tangy, Wanly

page 283: What's the Animal?
1. Count sheep
2. Cold duck *(Fish and turkey are also correct.)*
3. Play possum
4. Eat crow
5. Loan shark
6. Dark horse

page 284: It's All in the Name
1. Tan + Yahoo + Amin + Net + Bench
   Benjamin Netanyahu
2. Cone + Are + Oil + Thur + And
   Arthur Conan Doyle
3. E + It + Hair + Man + Tub
   Harriet Tubman

page 285: One-Minute Madness: Countries with Two-Word Names
(Other correct answers are possible.)
The Bahamas, Burkina Faso, Costa Rica, Cote d'Ivoire, Czech Republic, Dominican Republic, East Timor, El Salvador, Equatorial Guinea, The

Gambia, Guinea-Bisseau, Marshall Islands, New Zealand, North Korea, St. Lucia, San Marino, Saudi Arabia, Sierra Leone, Solomon Islands, South Africa, South Korea, South Sudan, Sri Lanka, United Kingdom, United States, Vatican City

page 286: Syllability

1. Curiosity
   CU • RI • OS • I • TY
2. Pancake
   PAN • CAKE
3. Popcorn
   POP • CORN
4. Screwdriver
   SCREW • DRI • VER
5. Vitamin
   VI • TA • MIN
6. Arithmetic
   A • RITH • ME • TIC
7. Dictionary
   DIC • TION • AR • Y
8. Newscaster
   NEWS • CAST • ER
9. Unveil
   UN • VEIL

Page 288: Eights & Fours

(Other correct answers are possible.)
1. Calendar   Card/Lane
2. Fracture   Turf/Race

page 289: Secret Word: Spaghetti

(Other correct answers are possible.)
4 Letters: Ages, Apes, Apse, East, Eats, Gait, Gape, Gaps, Gash, Gasp, Gate, Gets, Gist, Hags, Hasp, Hate, Hats, Heap, Heat, Hips, Hits, Page, Past, Path, Pats, Peas, Peat, Pegs, Pest, Pets, Pies, Pigs, Pita, Pits, Sage, Seat, Shag, Ship, Sigh, Site, Spat, Spit, Stag, Step, Tags, Tape, Taps, Teas, Teat, Test, That, This, Ties, Tips, Tits

5 Letters: Eight, Gaits, Gapes, Gates, Haste, Hates, Heaps, Heats, Heist, Pages, Paste, Paths, Phase, Pitas, Sepia, Shape, Sight, Spate, Spite, Stage, State, Tapes, Taste, Teats, **Tight *****, Tithe

*** Secret Word

page 290: Griddle

(Other correct answers are possible.)
4 Letters: Able, Alee, Bade, Bald, Bale, Bate, Bead, Beat, Beet, Bled, Dale, Data, Date, Deal, Deed, Dele, Ding, Dint, Dong, Geed, Idea, Iota, Late, Lead, Node, Tale, Teal, Teat, Teed, Toad, Toed, Tong

5 Letters: Abate, Baled, Bated, Baton, Blade, Bleat, Bleed, Dated, Deled, Dingo, Elate, Ingot, Table

6 Letters: Delete, Dinged, Elated, Indeed, Lading, Tabled, Tonged

7 Letters: Belated, Bleated, Deeding, Leading

8 Letters: Bleeding

page 293: Word Tower
(Other correct answers are possible.)
1. Do
2. Dog
3. Dock
4. Dozen
5. Double
6. Dolphin
7. Document
8. Dormitory

page 294: Odd Man Out
1. *Felix* is the odd man out. All the rest are entertainment awards.
2. *Trident* is the odd man out. All the rest are internet websites.
3. *Toronto* is the odd man out. All the others are names of the Great Lakes.
4. *Shrimp* is the odd man out. All the others are things you count.

page 295: Say What?
1. No man is an island.
2. The early bird catches the worm.
3. Actions speak louder than words.
4. Easy come, easy go.
5. Better late than never.

page 296: Counting Syllables
(In some cases, other correct answers are possible.)
1. April, July, August
2. Argentina, Bolivia, Colombia
3. Bean, Beet, Chard, Corn, Kale, Leek, Pea, Squash, Yam
4. Bush (George H. W.), Bush (George W.), Ford, Grant, Hayes, Pierce, Polk, Taft, Trump

page 297: Riddle Me This
When it's not raining.

page 298: Happy Endings
1. **Ger**   Anger, Badger, Finger, Swinger
2. **Oke**   Coke, Smoke, Stroke, Provoke
3. **Lop**   Gallop, Wallop, Develop, Scallop
4. **Und**   Pound, Refund, Compound, Profound

page 299: Two by Three
(Other correct answers are possible.)
L   Leek/Lettuce, Lewis/Larry, Lexus/Lincoln
O   Okra/Onion, Orson/Oliver, Oldsmobile/Opel
P   Parsnip/Potato, Peter/Phillip, Pontiac/Plymouth

page 300: Number Words

1. Car2n   Cartoon
2. S10ch   Stench
3. Qui9   Quinine
4. 4est   Forest
5. Or8or   Orator

page 301: Fill In the Letters

(Other correct answers are possible.)

1. Mica, Mice, Mien, Miff, Mike, Mild, Mile, Milk, Mill, Mime, Mind, Mine, Mini, Mink, Mint, Minx, Mire, Miso, Miss, Mist, Mite, Mitt
2. Aught, Eight, Fight, Light, Might, Night, Ought, Right, Sight, Tight

page 302: Do the Math!

1. 1 in 2. (There are six sides/numbers to a die.)
2. 26 out of 52
3. 1 in 13 (4 out of 52)
4. They are equally likely. You have a 50-50 chance of tossing a coin and getting heads, and you have a 50-50 chance of pulling a red card from a deck of 52 cards.

page 303: Wacky Wordy

One step forward, two steps back

page 304: Sentence Sleuth

1. Canary **"can a ry**e . . . "
2. Falcon "of**fal," Con**nie said . . .
3. Raven "zeb**ra ven**tured . . ."

page 305: Double Trouble

1. Blind
2. Short
3. Test
4. Secret

page 306: Run the Alphabet: Sports

(Other correct answers are possible.)

Archery	Mountain biking
Badminton	Nordic skiing
Cricket	Polo
Diving	Quoits
Equestrian	Racquetball
Fishing	Skiing
Gymnastics	Tennis
Hockey	Ultimate frisbee
Ice skating	Volleyball
Judo	Wrestling
Karate	Yachting
Luge	

page 307: What's the Word?

Bra Cobra, Brain, Bravest, Bracelet
Eat Beat, Wheat, Breath, Creature
Ire Wired, Desire, Admire, Director
Get Budget, Nugget, Target, Vegetable

page 308: Riddle Me This

The maid. There is no mail delivery on Sundays.

page 309: **One-Minute Madness: Ten Largest US States (in area)**
Alaska, Texas, California, Montana, New Mexico, Arizona, Nevada, Colorado, Oregon, Wyoming

page 310: **Hidden Quotation**
1. Through, Queue, Clue, Flu, Gnu
2. BMW, Lexus, Kia, Lotus
3. UTI (urinary tract infection), BP (blood pressure)
4. Nescafé, Keurig, Folgers
5. Hopi, Apache, Cree

Quotation: We didn't lose the game; we just ran out of time.

page 312: **Give Me a Word That . . .**
(Other correct answers are possible.)
1. Bait, Chow, Doll, Exam, Full, Grim, Hazy, Iris, Jobs, Kick, Lynx, Mark, Oboe . . . *(Many, many other answers are possible.)*
2. Catalog, Catch, Category, Cater, Cathedral, Catnap, Catnip, Cattle
3. Bland, Command, Demand, Errand, Expand, Gland, Grand, Homeland, Husband, Inkstand, Island, Stand, Thousand, Wetland

page 313: **Picture Connections**
Things that come in fives: Fingers, Vowels, Olympic rings

Things with pockets: Pita bread, Pool table, Pants

Red: Cross, Buttons, Eye

Image Credits

(Cube); © Photoguerilla (Pickle); © Olaola12 (Letter P); © Liubomirt (Sheet Music); © Gerduess (Letter Z); © Michaelfair (Drum); © Draftmode (Apple); © Siberica27 (Paw); © Lineartist (Halo); © Sdbower (Military Jet); © Viter8| (Tick). Page 181: © Oleksandr Bilyi (Scottish Fold); © Scubabartek (Balaclava); © Ondřej Prosický (Kinkajou); © Mark Herreid (Spork); © Balipadma (Geoduck); © Sarawuth Somboun (F-Hole). Page 192: © Dmitry Zimin (Apron); © Difenbahia Difenbahi (Steak); © Smileus (Tree); © Rolmat (Car); © Vitali Enhelbrekht (Jack); © Anat Chantrakool (Butter); © Suwat Pattanawadee (Guitar); © Elisabeth Burrell (Kite); © Lianquan Yu (Elephant). Page 197: © Gawriloff (Knees); © Dio5050 (Saw); © Feng Yu (Key); © Koldunova Anna (Choke); © Aleksandar Kamasi (Cash); © Oleg Doroshin (Gum). Page 202: © Mohàmed Osama (Comb); © Phanuwatn (Letter B); © David Woods (Moon). Page 223: © Andreypolitov (Axe); © Ratselmeister (Letter L); © Iofoto (Meter); © Axel Bueckert (Number 8); © Martin Isaac (Plaid); © Igor Alferov (Doll); © Gerduess (Letter S); © Pamela Mcadams (Cents); © Chernetskaya (Abs); © Monika Wisniewska (Sewing); © Aleph Snc (Lute); © Carlos Caetano (Leaf) © Ratselmeister (Letter F). Page 236: © Sebastian (Window); © Thes2680 (Cowboy); © Georgsv (Treasure Chest); © Photographerlondon (Baby's Bottom); © Grigor Atanasov (Clock); © Vadym Nechyporenko (Tropical Island). Page 243: © Leiladraws (Lace); © Cheryl - Annette Parker (Swing); © Slobodan Tomic (Escape); © Üstün Ibisoglu (Stick Shift); © Dmitry Belyaev (Heel); © Geerati (Strike); © Jon Kroninger (Pull Tab); © Nataliia Prokofyeva (Tongue); © Teerawut Bunsom (Fly). Pages 256–257: © Jeeragone Inrut (Apple Core); © Anton Starikov (Cigarette); © Skypixel (School Bus); © Tina Zovteva (Cot); © Yael Weiss (King); © Vasile Bobirnac (China); © Valya82 (Coffee); © Amsis1 (Ski); © Axel Bueckert (Number 10); © Phanuwatn (Letter S); © Aje (Letter C); © Hpphoto (Fern); © Olaola12 (Letter F); © Vladimirfloyd (Knee). Page 262: © Wesley Abrams (Tent); © Anatol1973 (Deuce); © Aetmeister (Ant); © Planetfelicity (Planet); © Ninell (Ear); © Ruslanchik (Knot). Page 276: © Mnogosmyslov Aleksey (Paw); © Gerduess (Letters P, D, F, C); © Vaclav Volrab (Fence); © Ominaesi (Miner); © Richard Lammerts (Oar); © Ljupco (Mitt); © Aje (Letters M, P); © Palabra (Tees); © Antares614 (Can); © Tatjana Baibakova (Pawn); © Konstik (Swim); © Drohn88 (Knit); © Svetlana Kurochkina (Tea). Page 313: © Maryd15 (Cross); © Naiyanab (Olympic Rings); © Valentino2 (Eye); © Edwardgerges (Billiards); © Juan Moyano (Pita); © Marilyn Gould (Button); © Marcogovel (Vowels); © MilsiArt (Shorts); © Tasakorn Kongmoon (Fingers).

Public Domain: Page 43: Bob McNeely, The White House (Bill Clinton). Page 257: Gerald R. Ford Library (Gerald Ford).

About the Author

Nancy Linde created and runs Never2Old4Games.com, an online subscription service for activities professionals working with senior citizens at assisted living residences, retirement communities, senior centers, and other senior-serving organizations. She is also the author of *399 Games, Puzzles & Trivia Challenges Specially Designed to Keep Your Brain Young* and *417 More Games, Puzzles & Trivia Challenges Specially Designed to Keep Your Brain Young*. Prior to her work creating games for seniors, she was a filmmaker who produced, wrote, and directed more than a dozen documentary films, mostly for the PBS series *NOVA*. She lives in Massachusetts.

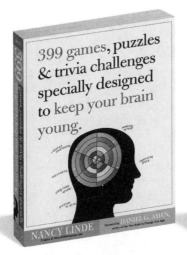
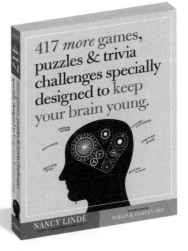